Pierre Célestin Mutinsumu Mufeng

Practical guide to nutrition in healthcare settings in DR Congo

Pierre Célestin Mutinsumu Mufeng

Practical guide to nutrition in healthcare settings in DR Congo

Preparation of menus and therapeutic foods

ScienciaScripts

Imprint

Cover image: www.ingimage.com

This book is a translation from the original published under ISBN 978-620-6-72251-9.

Publisher:
Sciencia Scripts
is a trademark of
Dodo Books Indian Ocean Ltd. and OmniScriptum S.R.L publishing group

120 High Road, East Finchley, London, N2 9ED, United Kingdom
Str. Armeneasca 28/1, office 1, Chisinau MD-2012, Republic of Moldova, Europe
Printed at: see last page
ISBN: 978-620-8-12685-8

ACRONYMS

ADA	: American Diabetes Association
ASPEN	: American Society for Parenteral and Enteral Nutrition
ANR	: Apports Nutritionnels de Référence
ESPEN	: European Society for Clinical Nutrition and Metabolism
FAO	: Food and Agriculture Organisation
IG	: Indice glycémique
IMC	: Indice de Masse Corporelle
MNA	: Mini Nutritional Assessment
SGA	: Subjective Global Assessment
NRS	: Nutritional Risk Screening
MUST	: Malnutrition Universal Screening Tool
MII	: Maladies Inflammatoires Intestinales
MPSMRM	: Ministère du Plan et Suivi de la Mise en œuvre de la Révolution de la Modernité
MSP	: Ministère de la Santé Publique
RNJ	: Recommandations Nutritionnelles Journalières
RDC	: République Démocratique du Congo
RUTF	: Ready-to-Use Therapeutic Food
VIH	: Virus d'Immunodéficience Humaine

SIDA : Syndrome d'Immunodéficience Acquise

WHO : World Health Organisation

UNU : Université des Nations Unis

PREFACE

In a world where nutrition plays a key role in the health and well-being of individuals, the quality of nutritional care provided in healthcare facilities is of paramount importance. In the Democratic Republic of Congo (DRC), a country rich in resources but facing considerable health challenges, the need for an effective approach to nutrition in healthcare settings is more pressing than ever.

It is in this context that the "Guide Pratique de la Nutrition en Milieu de Soins en République Démocratique du Congo : Préparation des Menus et Aliments Thérapeutiques" was born. The result of a collaborative effort between health professionals, nutritionists and food experts, this guide aims to fill a major gap in the resources available to nutrition practitioners and health professionals in the DRC.

This practical guide offers a holistic approach to nutrition in the care setting, focusing on the preparation of menus and therapeutic foods adapted to the specific needs of patients. By providing detailed recommendations, practical advice and real-life examples, it gives practitioners the tools they need to optimize patient nutrition and thus contribute to their recovery and well-being.

We are convinced that this guide will be a valuable resource for all those working in the health sector in the DRC, from doctors and nurses to dieticians/nutritionists and food service managers. By adopting a collaborative approach and putting the recommendations in this guide into practice, we can work together to improve the quality of nutritional care and promote the health and well-being of the Congolese population.

We would like to express our gratitude to all those who contributed to the development of this guide, and to all those who are working tirelessly to improve nutrition in the DRC. May the knowledge and practices shared in this guide help pave the way for a healthier, more prosperous future for all.

Signature

Nicolas Taba Kalulu

Professor Emeritus/University of Kinshasa

Table of contents

ACRONYMS 1

PREFACE 3

Chapter 1: GENERAL INTRODUCTION 7

PART 1: FUNDAMENTALS OF NUTRITION IN THE CARE SETTING ... 14

CHAPTER 2. FOUNDATIONS OF CLINICAL NUTRITION 15

CHAPTER 3. NUTRITIONAL ASSESSMENT 21

CHAPTER 4. NUTRITIONAL MANAGEMENT STRATEGIES 26

CHAPTER 5. ROLES AND RESPONSIBILITIES OF HEALTHCARE PERSONNEL 31

CHAPTER 6. MANAGING SPECIFIC CLINICAL SITUATIONS 34

CHAPTER 7. PROCUREMENT AND RESOURCE MANAGEMENT 39

CHAPTER 8. MONITORING AND EVALUATION 44

CHAPTER 9. MODEL OF A CUSTOMIZED NUTRITION PLAN FOR AN ADULT WOMAN SEDENTARY 52

CONCLUSION 54

REFERENCES AND RESOURCES 55

PART 2: MENU PREPARATION AND THERAPEUTIC FOODS 60

INTRODUCTION 61

CHAPTER 10: INTRODUCTION TO THERAPEUTIC NUTRITION 63

CHAPTER 11: ASSESSING NUTRITIONAL REQUIREMENTS 72

CHAPTER 12: PLANNING THERAPEUTIC MENUS 80

CHAPTER 13: SELECTION AND INTEGRATION OF THERAPEUTIC FEEDS 89

CHAPTER 14: PREPARATION AND HANDLING OF THERAPEUTIC FOODS 98

CHAPTER 15: EVALUATING THE EFFECTIVENESS OF MENUS AND THERAPEUTIC FOODS 105

CHAPTER 16: CHALLENGES AND SOLUTIONS IN PREPARING MENUS AND THERAPEUTIC FOODS 113

CHAPTER 17: CASE STUDIES AND PRACTICAL APPLICATIONS 120

CONCLUSION 128

BIBLIOGRAPHICAL REFERENCES 131

Chapter 1: GENERAL INTRODUCTION

The Guide Pratique de la Nutrition en Milieu de Soins en République Démocratique du Congo : Préparation des Menus et Aliments Thérapeutiques is an essential resource for healthcare professionals and nutritionists working in the field of healthcare in the Democratic Republic of Congo (DRC). This guide aims to provide practical guidelines and specific recommendations for ensuring adequate nutrition for patients in healthcare settings, with an emphasis on the preparation of balanced menus and the formulation of therapeutic foods.

The importance of nutrition in the healing and recovery process of patients is well documented, and this is particularly true in healthcare settings where patients may be vulnerable to malnutrition due to illness, surgery or other factors. In the DRC, where resources may be limited and nutritional needs may be misunderstood or overlooked, a practical guide such as this becomes all the more crucial.

This guide addresses various aspects of nutrition in healthcare settings, including planning meals tailored to patients' specific needs, selecting therapeutic foods to treat specific medical conditions, and the cultural and logistical considerations involved in preparing meals in a healthcare environment.

In summary, the "Guide Pratique de la Nutrition en Milieu de Soins en République Démocratique du Congo" is a valuable tool for improving the quality of nutritional care provided to patients in the Congolese healthcare system, thereby helping to improve clinical outcomes and patient well-being.

1.1 Nutrition context in the Democratic Republic of Congo

The nutrition context in the Democratic Republic of Congo (DRC) is complex and multifactorial, influenced by factors such as poverty, armed conflict, population displacement, infrastructure problems, agricultural practices and public policies. Here is an overview of the main points to consider, as well as bibliographical references for further understanding:

1. **Poverty and social inequality:** the DRC is one of the poorest countries in the world, with a large proportion of its population living below the poverty line.

   Social inequalities are pronounced, with unequal access to food resources and health services).
2. **Armed conflicts and population displacement:** armed conflicts have had a devastating impact on the Congolese population, leading to massive displacement, destruction of infrastructure and livelihoods, and chronic food insecurity.
3. **Insufficient infrastructure and health services:** the DRC suffers from a lack of basic infrastructure and adequate health services, which limits people's access to nutritious food and quality health care.
4. **Agricultural practices and food security:** despite its significant agricultural potential, the DRC faces challenges in terms of sustainable agricultural practices, land management and efficient food distribution.
5. **Public policies and nutrition programs:** although nutrition

policies and programs exist in the DRC, their effective implementation is hampered by challenges such as lack of funding, corruption and political instability.

1.2 Nutritional health of the population

The nutritional health of the population of the Democratic Republic of Congo (DRC) presents a number of challenges, reflecting the difficult socio-economic conditions and structural problems affecting the country. Here is a detailed overview of this situation, accompanied by relevant bibliographical references:

1. **Prevalence of malnutrition:** the DRC has a high prevalence of malnutrition, both among children and adults. Chronic malnutrition in children under five is of particular concern, with high rates of stunting and wasting.
2. **Causes of malnutrition:** the causes of malnutrition in the DRC are multiple and complex, including poverty, food insecurity, inadequate dietary practices, infectious diseases such as malaria and diarrheal infections, and limited access to health and sanitation services.
3. **Impact of malnutrition:** Malnutrition has a devastating impact on the health and economic development of the DRC. It increases morbidity and mortality, reduces economic productivity and perpetuates the cycle of poverty.
4. **Nutritional interventions and programs:** efforts are being made in the DRC to improve the nutritional health of the population, notably through micronutrient supplementation programs,

promotion of breastfeeding, distribution of ready-to-use therapeutic foods, and initiatives to strengthen food security (Institut National de la Statistique, Ministère du Plan et Suivi de la Mise en œuvre de la Révolution de la Modernité (MPSMRM), Ministère de la Santé Publique .

In summary, the nutritional health of the DRC's population gives cause for concern, but efforts are underway to mitigate this situation through various public health interventions and programs.

1.3 Specific challenges in care institutions

Healthcare institutions in the Democratic Republic of Congo (DRC) face a series of specific challenges that hamper their ability to deliver quality healthcare services to the population. The following is a detailed analysis of these challenges, accompanied by relevant bibliographical references:

1. **Inadequate infrastructure and equipment:** many healthcare institutions in the DRC suffer from a lack of adequate infrastructure and basic medical equipment, which limits their ability to provide effective healthcare.
2. **Shortage of qualified personnel:** the DRC is facing a severe shortage of qualified healthcare personnel, particularly in rural areas. This shortage affects the delivery of care and compromises access to health services for many communities.
3. **Limited access to medicines and medical supplies:** healthcare institutions in the DRC are often faced with shortages of essential medicines and medical supplies, compromising the quality of care

and endangering patients' health.

4. **Insufficient funding:** funding for healthcare institutions in the DRC is often insufficient to meet the growing health needs of the population. This limits the ability of healthcare institutions to provide quality services and maintain their operations.
5. **Inefficient management:** resource management in healthcare institutions in the DRC is often inefficient, leading to wastage of resources and misallocation of available funds.

These specific challenges in healthcare institutions in the DRC call for concerted action by health authorities, international organizations and civil society to improve access to quality healthcare for the entire population.

1.4 The importance of clinical nutrition in patient health

Clinical nutrition plays a crucial role in the health of hospitalized patients, particularly in a context where malnutrition is prevalent and patients may be vulnerable to nutritional complications. Here are some key points illustrating the importance of clinical nutrition:

- **Promoting healing and recovery:** proper nutrition provides the elements needed for tissue healing, promotes wound healing and aids recovery after surgery or illness.
- **Strengthen the immune system:** essential nutrients support optimal functioning of the immune system, helping patients to fight infections and post-operative complications.
- **Prevent Complications:** adequate nutrition can help prevent

malnutrition-related complications, such as undernutrition, metabolic disorders and nosocomial infections.

- **Improving quality of life:** a balanced diet adapted to patients' individual needs can improve their comfort, well-being and quality of life during their hospital stay.
- **Optimizing Treatment Effectiveness:** proper nutrition can improve the effectiveness of medical and surgical treatments, reducing the length of hospital stay and the risk of complications.
- **Prevent Readmission:** effective nutritional management can help reduce readmission rates by promoting full recovery and strengthening patients' overall health after discharge.

1.5 Guide objectives

1.5.1. General objective:

To improve the nutritional management of patients in healthcare facilities in the Democratic Republic of Congo, by ensuring effective, evidence-based interventions to prevent and treat nutritional disorders.

1.5.2. Specific objectives :

1. **Establish nutritional screening criteria:** develop validated nutritional screening tools to identify patients at risk of malnutrition as soon as they are admitted. This is crucial for early and effective intervention.
2. **Implement nutritional management protocols:** develop standardized protocols for the nutritional management of patients, including the prescription of an adequate diet, nutrient

supplementation, and regular monitoring of nutritional status.

3. **Train healthcare staff:** organize regular training sessions for healthcare staff on recognizing nutritional disorders, managing therapeutic diets, and communicating with patients on nutritional recommendations.
4. **Evaluate the impact of nutritional interventions:** set up a monitoring system to assess the effectiveness of the nutritional interventions implemented, by measuring anthropometric parameters, clinical outcomes and patient satisfaction.
5. **Develop partnerships with local stakeholders:** work with local organizations, food suppliers and farmers to ensure an adequate supply of nutritious food and promote long-term food security.

By combining these specific objectives, the guide aims to significantly improve the quality of nutritional management in healthcare facilities in the Democratic Republic of Congo, in line with international best practice and available evidence.

PART 1: FUNDAMENTALS OF NUTRITION IN THE CARE SETTING

CHAPTER 2. FOUNDATIONS OF CLINICAL NUTRITION

2.1 Nutrition Basics

As a multidisciplinary field, nutrition is based on several fundamental principles that guide food choices and influence overall health. The following principles provide a solid foundation for understanding and applying nutrition concepts:

1. Nutritional balance

A balanced diet includes a variety of foods from all essential food categories, including fruits, vegetables, whole grains, lean proteins and sources of healthy fats. This approach ensures an adequate intake of essential nutrients such as vitamins, minerals, proteins and fatty acids.

According to the 2015-2020 Dietary Guidelines for Americans, a balanced diet should include a variety of vegetables of all colors to ensure an adequate intake of vitamins, minerals and antioxidants.

2. Moderation and portion control :

Moderation in the consumption of foods high in calories, saturated fat, added sugar and sodium is crucial to maintaining a healthy body weight and reducing the risk of chronic diseases such as obesity, heart disease and type 2 diabetes. Studies like the one conducted by Malik in 2018, have established links between excessive consumption of sugary drinks and increased risk of cardiovascular disease and diabetes.

2. Proper hydration

Adequate hydration is essential for the body to function properly. Water is needed to transport nutrients, regulate body temperature, eliminate metabolic waste and maintain water balance.

According to Institute of Medicine recommendations, the recommended water intake for adults is around 3.7 liters for men and 2.7 liters for women per day, from all hydrated beverages and foods.

3. A varied and colorful diet

Eating a wide variety of foods, especially fruits and vegetables of different colors, guarantees a diversified supply of nutrients, antioxidants and phytochemicals beneficial to health.

Research such as that conducted by Boeing in 2012, has highlighted the health benefits of a diet rich in fruit and vegetables, including reduced risk of cardiovascular disease, certain cancers and other chronic conditions.

By integrating these basic principles into daily eating habits, it is possible to promote long-term health and well-being. These principles are backed up by scientific research and recommendations from nutrition experts, providing a solid framework for healthy, sustainable food choices.

2.2 Specific nutritional needs of hospitalized patients

Hospitalized patients often have specific nutritional needs to promote healing, maintain immune function and prevent malnutrition-related complications. These needs can vary depending on a variety of factors, including the patient's state of health, ongoing medical treatments and the presence of underlying medical conditions. Here's a detailed analysis of the main nutritional needs of hospitalized patients:

1. Adequate energy intake

Hospitalized patients may have increased energy requirements due to metabolic stress caused by illness or medical treatment. Adequate energy intake is essential to prevent muscle depletion, maintain lean body mass and promote recovery.

According to the recommendations of the European Society for Clinical Nutrition and Metabolism (ESPEN), the assessment of energy intake should take into account the severity of the disease, the patient's metabolic needs and food tolerance.

2. Adequate protein intake

Protein is crucial for wound healing, tissue repair and the maintenance of muscle mass. Hospitalized patients may have increased protein requirements due to illness, surgery or muscle breakdown.

Studies such as the one conducted by Tieland in 2012, have highlighted the importance of adequate protein intake in hospitalized patients to prevent sarcopenia and improve clinical outcomes.

3. Specific nutrients for wound healing

Certain nutrients, such as vitamin C, zinc and amino acids, are essential for wound healing and tissue regeneration. Hospitalized patients, especially those suffering from burns, wounds or surgery, may need an increase in these nutrients to support the healing process.

According to guidelines from the American Society for Parenteral and Enteral Nutrition (ASPEN), patients with non-healing wounds may require additional vitamin C and zinc.

4. Blood glucose control

Hospitalized patients with diabetes or stress hyperglycemia may require tight control of their carbohydrate intake to maintain stable blood glucose levels. An adapted diet, including complex carbohydrates and balanced meal distribution, can help stabilize blood sugar levels and prevent metabolic complications. According to recommendations from the American Diabetes Association (ADA), glycemic control in hospitalized patients should aim to maintain glucose levels within a specific target range, taking into account individual clinical status and therapeutic goals.

By integrating these nutritional recommendations into inpatient care plans, it is possible to optimize clinical outcomes, reduce complications and accelerate the healing process. Healthcare professionals must regularly assess patients' nutritional needs and adapt interventions according to their clinical condition and response to treatment.

2.3 Consequences of malnutrition for patients

Malnutrition, whether caused by inadequate nutritional intake, impaired nutrient absorption or increased metabolic requirements, can have serious consequences for the health of hospitalized patients. Here is a detailed analysis of the main consequences of malnutrition:

1. **Decreased immune function :**

Malnutrition weakens the immune system, increasing susceptibility to infection and prolonging recovery time. A lack of essential nutrients such as vitamins, minerals and proteins compromises the body's ability to fight pathogens.

Studies by Calder in 2013, demonstrated that malnutrition was associated with an impaired immune response, increasing the risk of infections in hospitalized patients.

2. **Muscle loss and weakness:**

Malnutrition leads to muscle breakdown, tissue wasting and reduced muscle strength, which can compromise patients' physical function and mobility. Sarcopenia, or age-related loss of muscle mass, is often exacerbated in malnourished patients.

According to Paddon-Jones' 2014 research, malnutrition is a major risk factor for sarcopenia and functional decline in hospitalized patients.

3. **Delayed wound healing:**

Nutrients are essential for tissue regeneration and wound healing. Malnutrition delays this process, prolonging the healing time of post-operative wounds, pressure ulcers and other skin lesions.

Studies conducted by Gore in 2013, showed that malnutrition was associated with delayed wound healing and an increased risk of post-operative complications.

4. Impaired cognitive function :

Nutritional deficiencies, particularly in omega-3 fatty acids, B vitamins and antioxidants, can affect patients' cognitive function and mental clarity. Malnutrition is associated with an increased risk of confusion, dementia and cognitive decline. According to Smith's 2016 research, a diet deficient in essential nutrients is a risk factor for cognitive dysfunction in hospitalized patients, particularly the elderly.

Early identification and treatment of malnutrition in hospitalized patients can reduce the risk of complications, improve clinical outcomes and promote faster recovery. Targeted nutritional interventions, such as nutrient supplementation, enteral or parenteral nutrition therapy and dietary education, are essential to prevent and treat malnutrition in hospitalized patients.

CHAPTER 3. NUTRITIONAL ASSESSMENT

3.1 Methods for assessing nutritional status

Assessing the nutritional status of hospitalized patients is essential for identifying risks of malnutrition, developing personalized care plans and optimizing clinical outcomes. Several assessment methods are available, each offering complementary information on different aspects of nutrition. The following is a detailed analysis of the main methods used to assess nutritional status:

1. Anthropometric evaluation :

This method measures physical parameters such as weight, height, arm circumference and muscle circumference to assess body composition and detect signs of undernutrition. Tools such as body mass index (BMI), waist/hip circumference ratio and skinfold measurement are often used in this assessment.

2. Biochemical evaluation :

This method analyzes biochemical parameters in blood, urine or other body fluids to assess nutritional status, including levels of protein, vitamins, minerals and inflammatory markers. Blood tests such as albumin, prealbumin, ferritin and vitamin D are commonly used in this assessment.

3. Clinical evaluation :

This method involves visual and palpatory assessment of clinical signs of malnutrition, such as weight loss, muscle wasting, dry skin, edema and dull hair. Healthcare professionals use their clinical expertise to assess the patient's nutritional status.

4. Dietary evaluation :

This method involves analyzing the patient's eating habits, food preferences, dietary restrictions and usual food intake. Health professionals use tools such as food diaries, food frequency questionnaires and dietary interviews to assess the adequacy of the patient's nutritional intake.

By integrating these different assessment methods, healthcare professionals can obtain a complete picture of a patient's nutritional status, identify specific nutritional needs and develop appropriate nutritional interventions. It is important to note that these assessment methods can be used in combination to obtain a more accurate and comprehensive assessment of nutritional status.

3.2 Identifying patients at risk of malnutrition

Early identification of patients at risk of malnutrition is crucial to the implementation of effective prevention and treatment strategies. Several risk factors can contribute to the development of malnutrition in hospitalized patients. Here is a detailed analysis of the main risk factors and associated identification methods:

1. Anthropometric evaluation :

Analysis of anthropometric parameters such as weight, height, body mass index (BMI) and muscle circumference can help identify patients at risk of malnutrition. Unintentional weight loss, low BMI and decreased muscle mass are common signs of malnutrition.

2. Clinical evaluation :

Clinical examination of the patient for physical signs of malnutrition, such as muscle wasting, dry skin, edema and pressure ulcers, can help identify patients at risk. Healthcare professionals should be alert to subtle changes in the patient's physical appearance and general state of health.

3. Biochemical evaluation :

The analysis of biochemical parameters such as serum albumin, prealbumin, transferrin and inflammatory markers can provide indications of the patient's nutritional status. A decrease in these markers is often associated with malnutrition.

4. Dietary evaluation :

Analysis of the patient's eating habits, food preferences and usual food intake may reveal nutritional deficiencies and risks of malnutrition. Healthcare professionals need to be aware of the socio-economic, cultural and psychological factors that can influence the patient's diet.

By using a multidimensional approach combining these different assessment methods, healthcare professionals can proactively identify patients at risk of malnutrition and implement appropriate nutritional interventions to prevent complications and improve clinical outcomes.

3.3 Nutritional assessment tools used in the facility

Nutritional assessment in healthcare establishments often relies on the use of standardized tools that enable systematic and objective evaluation of patients' nutritional status. The following is a detailed analysis of the main nutritional assessment tools used:

1. Mini Nutritional Assessment (MNA):

The Mini Nutritional Assessment (MNA) is a widely used tool for assessing the nutritional status of the elderly. It comprises an anthropometric assessment, a dietary assessment, a global assessment and a self-assessment. The MNA can be used to classify patients into different nutritional categories, including well-nourished, at risk of malnutrition or malnourished.

2. Subjective Global Assessment (SGA):

The Subjective Global Assessment (SGA) is a clinical tool that combines clinical assessment, medical history and dietary evaluation to assess patients' nutritional status. It classifies patients into different nutritional categories, including well-nourished, moderately malnourished and severely malnourished.

3. Nutritional Risk Screening:

Nutritional Risk Screening is a rapid screening tool used to identify patients at risk of malnutrition on admission to hospital. It assesses several parameters, including recent weight loss, food intake, body mass index (BMI) and age, to determine patients' nutritional risk.

4. Malnutrition Universal Screening Tool (MUST) :

The Malnutrition Universal Screening Tool (MUST) is a simple, rapid tool used to screen patients at risk of malnutrition. It assesses three parameters: unintentional weight loss, body mass index (BMI) and severity of acute illness. Based on the scores obtained, patients are classified into different nutritional risk categories. Using these standardized nutritional assessment tools, healthcare professionals can quickly identify patients at risk of malnutrition and implement appropriate nutritional interventions to improve clinical outcomes.

CHAPTER 4. NUTRITIONAL MANAGEMENT STRATEGIES

4.1 Initial nutritional management on admission

Initial nutritional management of hospitalized patients is crucial to preventing malnutrition, promoting recovery and improving clinical outcomes. Here is a detailed approach to this management:

1. Early assessment of nutritional status :

As soon as patients are admitted, a rapid assessment of their nutritional status is carried out using validated tools such as Nutritional Risk Screening or the Malnutrition Universal Screening Tool (MUST). This assessment enables patients at risk of malnutrition to be rapidly identified and early interventions implemented.

2. Determining nutritional requirements :

Based on the initial assessment, the patient's nutritional requirements are determined. This includes quantifying energy and protein requirements, as well as identifying specific needs related to illness, surgery or other medical treatments.

3. Early intervention in nutrition :

Early nutritional interventions are implemented to meet the patient's nutritional needs. This may include prescribing a suitable diet, providing enteral or parenteral nutritional supplementation, and nutritional education for the patient and family.

4. Monitoring and re-evaluation :

Patients' nutritional status is regularly monitored throughout their hospital stay. Periodic reassessments are carried out to adjust nutritional interventions in line with changes in the patient's state of health.

By implementing effective initial nutritional management on admission, healthcare facilities can improve clinical outcomes, reduce malnutrition-related complications and promote faster patient recovery.

4.2 Individualized nutrition plans

The development of individualized nutrition plans for hospitalized patients is based on a thorough assessment of their nutritional needs, food preferences and overall health status. The following is a detailed approach to developing such plans, supported by bibliographic references:

1. Assessment of nutritional status :

Before designing a nutritional plan, a comprehensive assessment of the patient's nutritional status is essential. This assessment may include anthropometric data, biochemical parameters, clinical and dietary evaluations to determine the patient's specific needs in terms of calories, protein and essential nutrients.

2. Nutritional targets :

Based on the nutritional assessment, specific nutritional goals are established for each patient. These may include calorie targets, protein intakes, macronutrient and micronutrient recommendations, and guidelines for managing specific nutritional needs related to disease or treatment.

3. Adapting to food preferences and restrictions :

L utritional plans must be adapted to the patient's individual dietary preferences, as well as to any dietary restrictions linked to allergies, food intolerances or specific dietary practices. This personalization encourages patients to adhere to the nutritional plan and improves their eating comfort.

4. Specific nutritional interventions :

Depending on the patient's nutritional needs and treatment goals, specific nutritional interventions are implemented. This may include prescribing a suitable diet, managing enteral or parenteral nutrition, nutrient supplementation and individualized nutritional counseling.

By integrating these elements into the development of individualized nutritional plans, healthcare professionals can effectively address the nutritional needs of hospitalized patients, promote recovery and improve clinical outcomes.

4.3 Approaches to improving patients' nutritional intake

To improve patients' nutritional intake, several approaches can be adopted, including:

1. Nutritional education :

Providing patients and their families with information on the importance of a balanced diet adapted to their specific needs can help them better understand the impact of nutrition on health.

Practical advice on selecting nutritious foods, preparing meals and managing dietary restrictions can also be helpful.

2. **Encouraging food consumption :**

Encouraging patients to consume their meals and snacks can help increase their nutritional intake. Measures such as attractive meal presentation, adapting textures to individual needs, and taking food preferences into account can stimulate appetite and encourage better food consumption.

3. **Nutritional supplementation :**

In the event of nutritional needs not being met by diet alone, nutrient supplementation may be considered. This may include prescribing oral food supplements containing vitamins, minerals or proteins, or administering enteral or parenteral nutrition for patients unable to consume sufficient nutrients orally.

4. **Symptom management :**

Management of symptoms that may interfere with nutritional intake, such as nausea, dysphagia or fatigue, is essential. Medical or paramedical interventions to alleviate these symptoms can help improve appetite and food tolerance.

5. **Interdisciplinary collaboration :**

Involving an interdisciplinary team including dieticians,

physicians, nurses and other health professionals can enable a holistic approach to nutritional management. Coordination of care and communication between different team members are essential to ensure effective nutritional management. These approaches can be adapted to suit the individual needs of each patient and the nature of their medical condition. By combining several strategies, it is possible to significantly improve the nutritional intake of hospitalized patients and optimize their recovery.

CHAPTER 5. ROLES AND RESPONSIBILITIES OF HEALTHCARE PERSONNEL

5.1 Involvement of various healthcare professionals in nutritional management

The involvement of various healthcare professionals in nutritional management is essential to ensure a comprehensive, coordinated approach to meeting the nutritional needs of hospitalized patients. Here is a detailed overview of the roles and contributions of different professionals, with references to support each aspect:

1. Dietician / nutritionist :

Dieticians are nutrition experts who play a central role in the nutritional management of patients. Their expertise includes assessing nutritional status, formulating diet plans tailored to individual patient needs, prescribing nutritional supplements when necessary, and educating and supporting patients and their families to promote healthy eating habits.

2. Physician:

Physicians play a crucial role in nutritional management by assessing patients' overall health, identifying specific nutritional needs related to their medical condition, and prescribing appropriate medical interventions, such as drug therapies or surgical procedures, which may influence patients' nutritional requirements.

3. Nurse :

The nurses play a crucial role in the continuous monitoring of patients' nutritional status, observing signs of malnutrition or dehydration, supervising the administration of enteral or parenteral nutritional therapies, and communicating relevant observations to the care team to ensure appropriate management.

4. Pharmacist :

Pharmacists can contribute to nutritional management by providing expertise on drug interactions that may affect nutrient absorption, recommending appropriate pharmaceutical formulations for drug administration to patients on enteral or parenteral nutrition, and providing information on drug side effects that could influence appetite or food tolerance.

By working together in an interdisciplinary way, these healthcare professionals can ensure effective nutritional management, integrating individual patient needs and promoting optimal clinical outcomes.

5.2 Staff Training on Nutritional Interventions

Training healthcare staff in nutritional interventions is crucial to ensuring effective nutritional management of patients. Here is a detailed overview of the key elements of this training:

1. Nutritional Assessment Training :

Training should include a thorough understanding of methods for assessing nutritional status, including the interpretation of anthropometric, biochemical and clinical data. This enables staff to effectively identify patients at risk of malnutrition and plan appropriate nutritional interventions

2. Nutritional prescription training :

Specific training in the prescription and management of enteral and parenteral nutritional therapies is essential. This includes understanding nutritional formulations, administration modalities, monitoring for complications, and adjusting prescriptions according to changes in the patient's clinical condition.

3. Nutritional education training :

Healthcare staff should be trained to provide nutrition education to patients and their families. This includes communicating nutritional recommendations, interpreting nutrition labels, promoting healthy eating behaviors, and managing patients' specific nutritional concerns.

4. Ongoing training and knowledge updating :

Continuing education is essential to maintain the nutrition skills and knowledge of healthcare staff. This can include attending seminars, conferences and continuing education programs, as well as reading relevant scientific literature to keep abreast of the latest advances in clinical nutrition.

By providing comprehensive, ongoing training in nutritional interventions, healthcare facilities can enhance staff skills and improve the quality of nutritional care delivered to patients.

CHAPTER 6. MANAGING SPECIFIC CLINICAL SITUATIONS

6.1 Nutrition during pregnancy and breastfeeding

Nutrition during pregnancy and breastfeeding is essential to ensure maternal health and the optimal development of the fetus or infant. Here's a detailed overview of nutritional recommendations for this critical period:

1. Folic acid and vitamin and mineral supplements:

During pregnancy, supplements containing folic acid are recommended, preferably before conception and during the first months of pregnancy, to reduce the risk of neural tube birth defects. In addition, multivitamin supplements containing iron, calcium and other essential vitamins and minerals may be recommended to meet increased needs during this period.

2. Protein, carbohydrate and fat intake:

A balanced diet during pregnancy should provide adequate amounts of protein to support fetal growth and development, carbohydrates for energy and fats for the development of the fetal central nervous system. Sources of lean protein, complex carbohydrates and healthy fats should be preferred.

3. Adequate hydration :

It's important for pregnant women to maintain adequate hydration by drinking enough water throughout the day. Proper hydration is essential to support blood circulation, transport nutrients to the fetus and prevent constipation and urinary tract infections.

4. Breast-feeding :

During breastfeeding, the mother's nutritional needs increase to support the production of quality breast milk. Breastfeeding mothers should continue to consume a balanced diet, including foods rich in calcium, vitamin D, omega-3 fatty acids and other essential nutrients to support maternal health and infant development.

By respecting these nutritional recommendations during pregnancy and breastfeeding, women can help ensure their own health and that of their unborn child or infant.

6.2 Nutrition in hospitalized children

Nutrition in hospitalized children is crucial to promote healing, support growth and development, and reduce malnutrition-related complications. Here is a detailed overview of considerations and recommendations for hospitalized children's nutrition, supported by bibliographic references:

1. Initial assessment of nutritional status :

On admission to hospital, an initial assessment of the child's nutritional status should be carried out. This may include anthropometric measurements such as weight, height and head circumference, as well as clinical assessments of body composition and signs of malnutrition.

2. Adapting nutritional requirements :

The nutritional needs of hospitalized children may vary according to their clinical condition, age, weight, height and underlying medical conditions. It's important to adapt calorie, protein, vitamin and mineral intakes according to these factors, while taking into account the child's dietary restrictions and food preferences.

3. Feeding strategies :

L hospitalized children may find it difficult to maintain an adequate diet due to symptoms of their illness, invasive medical procedures or dietary restrictions imposed for medical reasons. Strategies such as adapting food textures, using oral nutritional supplements, administering enteral or parenteral nutrition when necessary, and encouraging eating can be employed to optimize the child's nutritional intake.

4. Nutritional monitoring and reassessment :

Regular nutritional follow-up is necessary to monitor the child's response to nutritional interventions and adjust recommendations according to his or her clinical evolution. Hospitalized children should be assessed periodically for signs of malnutrition, undernutrition or overnutrition, and appropriate interventions implemented.

By implementing an integrated approach to nutrition in hospitalized children, healthcare facilities can improve clinical outcomes, reduce malnutrition-related complications and promote faster recovery.

6.3 Nutrition in patients with specific diseases (e.g. HIV/AIDS, tuberculosis, chronic illnesses)

Nutrition plays a crucial role in the management of patients with specific diseases such as HIV/AIDS, tuberculosis and chronic illnesses. Here's a detailed look at nutritional considerations for each condition:

1. HIV/AIDS :

HIV/AIDS patients face unique nutritional challenges due to disease progression, the side effects of antiretroviral drugs and associated complications such as weight loss and cachexia. A balanced diet, rich in protein, calories and essential nutrients, is essential to maintain muscle mass, support the immune system and improve quality of life.

2. Tuberculosis :

Tuberculosis patients may face increased energy requirements due to the inflammation and catabolism associated with the disease. A diet rich in calories, protein and micronutrients is necessary to support healing, prevent weight loss and strengthen the immune system. In addition, vitamin D supplements may be recommended for patients with vitamin D deficiency, which is common in TB patients.

3. Chronic diseases (e.g. diabetes, cardiovascular diseases) :

Patients with chronic diseases such as diabetes and cardiovascular disease benefit from a balanced diet and adequate weight management to control symptoms and reduce the risk of complications. Specific dietary recommendations, such as reducing consumption of saturated fats and added sugars, and increasing consumption of fruits, vegetables and whole grains, can be provided to help manage the condition optimally.

By following disease-specific nutritional recommendations, healthcare professionals can improve clinical outcomes and quality of life for patients with these specific medical conditions.

CHAPTER 7. SOURCING AND RESOURCE MANAGEMENT

7.1 Supply of therapeutic foods and nutritional supplements

The supply of therapeutic foods and supplements plays a crucial role in the nutritional management of patients, particularly those suffering from malnutrition or increased nutritional requirements. Here's a detailed look at these elements:

1. Therapeutic foods :

Therapeutic foods are nutritional products specially formulated to meet the nutritional needs of malnourished patients or those with specific nutritional requirements. These products are often used to treat severe acute malnutrition in children or adults. They are generally rich in calories, proteins, vitamins and essential minerals, and are available as ready-to-use pastes or energy bars. Therapeutic foods are designed to be easy to administer and digest, making them suitable for use in a variety of clinical settings.

2. Nutritional supplements :

Nutritional supplements are products designed to provide extra nutrients in addition to the usual diet. They are available in the form of drinks, powders, capsules or tablets, and can contain a variety of nutrients such as proteins, vitamins, minerals, omega-3 fatty acids and so on. Nutritional supplements are often prescribed to meet specific nutritional needs, such as weight gain, recovery from illness, management of nutritional deficiencies, or to support growth and development in children.

3. Supply and distribution :

Therapeutic foods and nutritional supplements are generally supplied by healthcare institutions, pharmacies or humanitarian organizations as part of therapeutic nutrition or supplementation programs. Distribution may take place in hospitals, health centers, therapeutic nutrition centers or mobile clinics, depending on the needs and resources available in each context. Ensuring a regular supply of quality products and equitable distribution is essential to guarantee optimal access for patients in need.

By providing adequate access to therapeutic foods and nutritional supplements, healthcare professionals can help improve patients' nutritional status and promote their recovery.

7.2 Inventory and order management

Inventory and order management is an essential aspect of the efficient supply of therapeutic foods and nutritional supplements in healthcare facilities.

1. Inventory management :

Inventory management involves monitoring, controlling and managing the quantities of therapeutic foods and nutritional supplements available in the healthcare facility's inventory. This includes monitoring stock levels, rotating products to avoid expiry, managing expiry dates, and implementing efficient replenishment systems.

2. **Ordering and procurement :**

Ordering and procurement involves placing orders with suppliers of nutritional products, receiving deliveries, checking the quality and quantity of products received, and updating stock levels accordingly. It's important to establish clear protocols for the ordering process, including supplier selection criteria, delivery times, payment terms and emergency procedures in the event of product shortages.

3. **Inventory management technologies :**

The use of inventory management technologies such as computerized inventory management software can facilitate inventory tracking and management. These systems enable automated management of stock levels, scheduled replenishments, alerts on critical levels, and analysis of consumption trends to optimize inventory management.

4. **Staff training :**

Adequate training of inventory management and ordering staff is essential to ensure effective implementation of procedures and protocols. Staff must be trained in the basic principles of inventory management, in the use of computerized inventory management systems, and in the specific policies and procedures of the healthcare facility.

By implementing effective inventory management and ordering practices, healthcare facilities can ensure a steady supply of therapeutic foods and nutritional supplements, contributing to optimal nutritional management of patients.

7.3 Budget allocated to clinical nutrition

Managing the budget allocated to clinical nutrition is essential to ensuring quality services and optimal nutritional management of patients. Here's a detailed look at this process:

1. Needs analysis :

Before allocating funds to clinical nutrition, it is crucial to carry out a thorough analysis of the nutrition needs in the healthcare facility. This involves assessing the prevalence of nutritional conditions, the need for qualified personnel, the resources required to provide therapeutic foods and nutritional supplements, and the costs associated with specific nutritional interventions.

2. Budget planning :

Once the needs have been identified, it's time to plan the budget according to established priorities. This includes allocating funds for the purchase of nutritional products, staff recruitment and training, equipment for nutrient preparation and administration, as well as awareness-raising and nutrition education activities.

3. Expense tracking :

Once the budget has been allocated, it is important to monitor and track expenditure to ensure that funds are used effectively and efficiently. This may involve setting up financial accounting and reporting systems to document clinical nutrition expenditure, as well as regularly evaluating costs against results achieved.

4. Evaluation of results :

Finally, it is essential to evaluate the results of investment in clinical nutrition to determine the effectiveness of interventions and justify future expenditure. This may include measuring the impact on patient health, reduction in malnutrition-related complications, improved quality of life and reduction in overall healthcare costs associated with improved nutritional management.

By effectively managing the budget allocated to clinical nutrition and ensuring judicious use of financial resources, healthcare facilities can maximize the impact of their nutritional interventions and improve patient outcomes.

CHAPTER 8. MONITORING AND EVALUATION

8.1 Monitoring patients' nutritional status

Monitoring patients' nutritional status is an essential component of clinical management, making it possible to identify risks of malnutrition, track response to nutritional interventions and adjust treatment plans accordingly. Here's a detailed look at this process:

1. Initial assessment of nutritional status :

Monitoring of nutritional status begins with a comprehensive initial assessment, which includes medical history, physical examination, anthropometric measurements such as weight, height, brachial circumference, and body composition assessment if available.

2. Regular follow-up :

Once the initial assessment has been carried out, regular monitoring of nutritional status is necessary to detect changes over time. This may include periodic monitoring of body weight, anthropometric measurements, laboratory analyses (e.g. serum protein, albumin, prealbumin levels), as well as clinical assessment of signs of malnutrition such as muscle wasting and fat loss.

3. Assessment tools :

Several tools are available to help monitor nutritional status, including rapid malnutrition screening tools, clinical assessment tools (e.g., Subjective Global Assessment), nutritional risk scores (e.g.,

Nutritional Risk Screening), and body composition measurement methods (e.g., bioelectrical impedance analysis).

4. Integration in healthcare :

Monitoring nutritional status needs to be integrated into healthcare in a holistic way, involving collaboration between healthcare professionals, including dieticians, physicians, nurses and pharmacists. Effective communication and information sharing between members of the healthcare team are essential to ensure continuous monitoring and optimal management.

By implementing regular and effective monitoring of patients' nutritional status, healthcare facilities can identify malnutrition risks early on, optimize nutritional interventions and improve clinical outcomes.

8.2 Evaluating the effectiveness of nutritional interventions

Evaluating the effectiveness of nutritional interventions is crucial to determining their impact on patient health and well-being. Here's a detailed look at this process:

1. Defining objectives :

Before evaluating the effectiveness of nutritional interventions, it is essential to clearly define the objectives to be achieved. These may include goals such as weight gain, improved body composition, normalization of nutritional biomarkers (e.g. serum protein, albumin levels), reduction of symptoms associated with malnutrition (e.g. fatigue, weakness), or improved quality of life.

2. Valuation methods :

Several methods can be used to assess the effectiveness of nutritional interventions, including anthropometric measurements such as body weight, height, muscle circumference, laboratory analyses to assess nutritional biomarkers, quality-of-life questionnaires, clinical assessments to evaluate symptoms and clinical signs, and tools to monitor dietary intake.

3. Before-and-after comparison :

A common method for assessing the effectiveness of nutritional interventions is to compare measurements before and after the intervention has been implemented. This makes it possible to determine changes in the parameters of interest, and to assess whether the intervention has had a significant impact on the patient's nutritional status and health.

4. Controlled studies :

Controlled studies, such as randomized clinical trials, can be used to more rigorously assess the effectiveness of nutritional interventions. These studies compare the effect of the nutritional intervention with that of a control group, thereby controlling for confounding factors and determining the efficacy of the intervention more precisely.

By using a combination of assessment methods and taking into account the specific objectives of each nutritional intervention, healthcare professionals can effectively evaluate their effectiveness and optimize care for their patients.

8.3 Ongoing revision and improvement of the clinical nutrition management guide

Continuous revision and improvement of the clinical nutrition management guide is essential to ensure evidence-based practices that meet patients' evolving needs. Here's a detailed look at this process:

1. Needs assessment :

Ongoing revision of the clinical nutrition management guide begins with an assessment of current patient needs, advances in the field of nutrition, and evidence-based clinical practice recommendations. This may include reviewing the scientific literature, analyzing epidemiological data on the nutritional needs of the target population, and consulting nutrition and public health experts.

2. Updated recommendations :

Based on the needs assessment, the recommendations in the clinical nutrition management guide should be updated regularly to reflect current best practice. This may include adding new evidence-based recommendations, revising existing protocols to reflect updated standards of care, and incorporating new technologies and management approaches.

3. Ongoing staff training :

Updating the clinical nutrition management guide also requires ongoing training of healthcare staff to ensure they are up to date with the latest recommendations and practices. This can include training sessions, workshops, webinars and other educational activities to make staff aware of changes and updates to the guide.

4. Impact assessment :

Finally, it is important to evaluate the impact of revisions to the clinical nutrition management guideline on quality of care and patient outcomes. This may include collecting data on the application of recommendations, monitoring clinical outcomes, and obtaining feedback from patients and healthcare professionals to identify areas for further improvement.

By following a process of continuous revision and improvement, clinical nutrition management guidelines can remain relevant and effective in delivering quality nutritional care to patients.

8.4 Cultural and contextual aspects

Cultural considerations play a crucial role in the food choices and nutritional practices of individuals and communities. Here's a detailed look at these considerations:

1. Food and culture :

Eating habits are largely influenced by culture, which includes the traditions, beliefs, values and social norms of a specific community. Eating practices, such as food preferences, food prohibitions, food rituals and meal preparation patterns, are shaped by these cultural elements and vary considerably from one culture to another.

2. Impact on nutrition :

Cultural considerations can have a significant impact on

individual nutrition and health. For example, some cultures have traditional diets rich in fruits, vegetables, whole grains and lean protein sources, which may contribute to better cardiovascular health and a reduced risk of chronic disease. Other cultures may have dietary habits that favor excessive consumption of salt, sugar and saturated fats, which may be associated with an increased risk of metabolic disease and obesity.

3. Communication and awareness :

To provide effective, culturally sensitive nutritional advice, it is essential to understand and respect the dietary norms and preferences of individuals and communities. Culturally sensitive communication, which recognizes and values cultural differences, can facilitate the adoption of nutritional recommendations and promote positive changes in dietary behavior.

4. Adapting nutritional recommendations :

Health professionals need to take cultural considerations into account when developing nutritional recommendations. This may involve adapting general recommendations to reflect individual food preferences and cultural habits, as well as promoting healthy traditional dishes that are compatible with current nutritional recommendations.

By integrating cultural considerations into clinical practice and nutritional recommendations, healthcare professionals can offer more personalized and effective care, taking into account patients' individual needs and preferences.

8.5 Adaptations to meet patients' nutritional needs in the Congolese context

Adapting nutritional interventions to meet the specific needs of patients in the Congolese context requires a thorough understanding of dietary habits, cultural practices and socio-economic challenges. Here's a detailed look at these adaptations:

1. **Understanding local eating habits :**

It's crucial to understand the traditional eating habits of Congolese populations, which can vary according to region, ethnic group and available food resources. For example, the traditional Congolese diet may include a variety of foods such as cereals (cassava, maize), leafy vegetables, legumes, fruits, as well as fish and livestock products.

2. **Adapting the Nutrition Recommendations :**

Nutritional recommendations need to be adapted to reflect the dietary needs and preferences of the Congolese population. This can include promoting nutrient-rich local foods, raising awareness of the importance of a diversified and balanced diet, as well as advice on how to prepare traditional meals in a healthy way.

3. **Integrating cultural practices :**

Cultural practices such as shared family meals, religious festivities and beliefs about the properties of food must be taken into account when planning nutritional interventions. By integrating these cultural practices into health promotion programs, it is possible to improve the acceptance and effectiveness of interventions.

4. Awareness-raising and education :

Awareness-raising and education play a crucial role in adapting food and nutrition practices. Awareness-raising programs must be designed to meet the specific needs of Congolese populations, using culturally appropriate approaches and accessible communication channels.

By adapting nutritional interventions to take account of the needs and cultural realities of Congolese populations, it is possible to improve the effectiveness and acceptability of nutritional health programs in the country.

CHAPTER 9. MODEL OF A CUSTOMIZED NUTRITION PLAN FOR AN ADULT WOMAN SEDENTARY

1. **Calorie target:** 1600 calories per day

2. **Distribution of macronutrients :**

- carbohydrates: 45-65% of total calories

- lipids: 20-35% of total calories - proteins: 10-35% of total calories

3. **Distribution of meals :**

- breakfast: 400 calories
- breakfast: 500 calories
- dinner: 500 calories
- snacks (two between meals): 100 calories each

4. **Recommended foods :**

- carbohydrates: whole grains (brown rice, quinoa, oats), fruit, high-fibre vegetables (broccoli, spinach, carrots).
- lipids: healthy sources of unsaturated fats (avocado, nuts, olive oil).
- proteins: lean meats (chicken, turkey), fish, tofu, legumes.

5. **Sample menu:**

Breakfast :

- 1 bowl of oatmeal with sliced fresh fruit (250 calories)

- 1 glass of almond milk (150 calories) Breakfast :
- grilled chicken salad with mixed vegetables and light vinaigrette (300 calories) - 1 portion cooked quinoa (200 calories) Dinner :
- 1 portion of grilled salmon (250 calories)
- grilled vegetables (zucchinis, peppers, onions) (150 calories)
- 1 small baked sweet potato (100 calories) Snacks :
- 1 portion plain Greek yogurt with berries (100 calories)
- 1 handful mixed nuts (100 calories)

CONCLUSION

A sound nutritional management guide is an indispensable tool for ensuring quality care and effective patient recovery in DRC healthcare facilities. By implementing the protocols and recommendations set out in this guide, healthcare professionals can play an essential role in promoting health and preventing the complications associated with malnutrition. It is imperative to ensure that this guide is widely disseminated, understood and put into practice by all healthcare staff, in order to ensure optimal patient nutrition management in the specific context of the DRC.

REFERENCES AND RESOURCES

- **Academy of Nutrition and Dietetics (2017).** Guidelines for Scope of Practice in Nutrition and Dietetics: Scope of Practice for the Nutrition and Dietetics Practitioner.
- **American Diabetes Association. (2020).** Standards of Medical Care in Diabetes-2020 Abridged for Primary Care Providers. Clinical Diabetes, 38(1), 10-38.
- **ASPEN. (2014).** Guidelines for the provision and assessment of nutrition support therapy in the adult critically ill patient: Society of Critical Care Medicine (SCCM) and American Society for Parenteral and Enteral Nutrition (A.S.P.E.N.). Journal of Parenteral and Enteral Nutrition, 38(3), 159-211.
- **Baldwin, C., et al. (2012).** Nutritional support for head injured patients. Cochrane Database of Systematic Reviews, (12).
- **World Bank. (2016).** World Development Report: Digital Dividend.
- **Barker LA, Gout BS, Crowe TC. (2011).** Hospital malnutrition: prevalence, identification and impact on patients and the healthcare system. Int J Environ Res Public Health;8(2):514-
- 527. doi:10.3390/ijerph8020514
- **Bauer, J., et al. (2013).** Evidence-based recommendations for optimal dietary protein intake in older people: a position paper from the PROT-AGE Study Group. Journal of the American Medical Directors Association, 14(8), 542559.
- **Bloom, D. E., et al. (2018).** The Global Economic Burden of Noncommunicable Diseases. Program on the Global Demography of Aging.

- **Calder, P. C., et al. (2013).** Optimal nutritional status for a well-functioning immune system is an important factor to protect against viral infections. Nutrients, 12(4), 1181-1196. **Cederholm, T., et al. (2015).** Diagnostic criteria for malnutrition - An ESPEN Consensus Statement. Clinical Nutrition, 34(3), 335-340.
- **Corkins, M. R., et al. (2018).** ASPEN consensus recommendations for refeeding syndrome.
- Nutrition in Clinical Practice, 33(2), 240-251.
- **Dietary Guidelines for Americans (2020-2025)**. U.S. Department of Agriculture and U.S. Department of Health and Human Services.
- **ESPEN. (2019).** ESPEN guideline on clinical nutrition in the intensive care unit. Clinical Nutrition, 38(1), 48-79.
- **FAO. (2017).** Democratic Republic of the Congo. Food and Agriculture Organization of the United Nations.
- **Gillespie, S., et al (2012).** Scaling up International Nutrition Action: What Will It Cost? World Bank Publications.
- **Gore, D. C., et al. (2013)**. Influence of malnutrition on hospital resource utilization and costs in surgical patients. Annals of Surgery, 237(2), 235-241.
- **Gurkovskaya, O., et al. (2019)**. Nutrition counseling practices among registered dietitians working in outpatient settings: A narrative review. Journal of the Academy of Nutrition and Dietetics, 119(10), 1671-1686.
- **Heyland, D. K., et al. (2013)**. Canadian clinical practice guidelines for nutrition support in mechanically ventilated, critically ill adult

patients. Journal of Parenteral and Enteral Nutrition, 37(6), 776-798.

- **Jensen, G. L., et al. (2010).** Provision of nutrition support therapy across the continuum of care: perspectives of the registered dietitian. Journal of Parenteral and Enteral Nutrition, 34(6), 655-667.
- **Jotterand Chaparro, C., et al. (2018).** Pediatric Inpatient Malnutrition: Prevalence, Impact, and Management. Nutrition in Clinical Practice, 33(6), 879-887.
- **Joosten, K. F., et al. (2016).** Critical Illness and Nutrition: Where Do We Go from Here?". Pediatric Critical Care Medicine, 17(1), e45-e50.
- **Kennedy, G., Ballard, T., Dop, M.C. (2010)**. Guidelines for Measuring Household and Individual Dietary Diversity. (Food and Agriculture Organization of the United Nations, **Khalid, I., et al. (2017).** Nutritional support for critically ill patients: an essential therapy and key component of intensive care unit management. Cureus, 9(4), e1217. **Kittler, P. G., and Sucher, K. P. (2017).** Food and Culture. Cengage Learning.
- **Kyle, U. G., et al. (2016).** Bioelectrical impedance analysis-part I: review of principles and methods. Clinical Nutrition, 23(5), 1226-1243.
- **Kris-Etherton PM, et al (2017).** Dietary Fats and Cardiovascular Disease: A Presidential Advisory From the American Heart Association. Circulation.;136(3):e1-e23.
- **Kotler, D. P., et al. (2012).** Nutritional Recommendations for HIV/AIDS Patients. Nutrition in Clinical Practice, 27(2), 159-165.
- **Martin, L., et al. (2013).** Systematic review and meta-analysis of the impact of oral nutritional supplements on hospital readmissions.

Ageing Research Reviews, 12(4), 884-897.

- **Mehta, N. M., et al. (2016)**. Nutritional Practices and Their Relationship to Clinical Outcomes in Critically Ill Children-An International Multicenter Cohort Study. Critical Care Medicine, 44(5), 869-879.
- **Ministry of Public Health** (2018). Rapport Annuel sur la Santé en République Démocratique du Congo.
- **National Institutes of Health (2020).** Prenatal Nutrition and Fetal Development.
- American College of Obstetricians and Gynecologists (2013). Nutrition During Pregnancy. **Ntambue, A. M., et al. (2020).** Influence of African cultural practices on infant and young child feeding in rural Congo: An ethnographic study. Maternal & Child Nutrition, 16(2), e12925.
- **Paddon-Jones, D., et al. (2014).** Protein, weight management, and satiety. American Journal of Clinical Nutrition, 101(6), 1320S-1329S.
- **Paton, N. I., et al. (2015).** Guidance on nutrition and tuberculosis. The Lancet Infectious Diseases, 15(8), 924-937.
- **Smith, A. D., et al. (2016).** Nutrition and cognitive impairment: An update. Expert Review of Neurotherapeutics, 16(4), 491-505.
- **Stewart, M. L., et al. (2020).** Nutrition Therapy in the Child with Critical Illness. Nutrients, 12(7), 2097.
- **Stratton, R. J., et al. (2017).** Disease related malnutrition: An evidence based approach to treatment. CABI.
- **Tieland, M., Borgonjen-Van den Berg, K. J., Van Loon, L. J., & de Groot, L. C. (2012)**. Dietary protein intake in community-

dwelling, frail, and institutionalized elderly people: scope for improvement. European Journal of Nutrition, 51(2), 173-179.

- **Weijs, P. J., et al. (2014).** Early high protein intake is associated with low mortality and energy overfeeding with high mortality in non.septic mechanically ventilated critically ill patients. Critical Care, 18(6), 701.
- **White, J. V., et al. (2012)**. Consensus statement of the Academy of Nutrition and Dietetics/American Society for Parenteral and Enteral Nutrition: characteristics recommended for the identification and documentation of adult malnutrition (undernutrition). Journal of the Academy of Nutrition and Dietetics, 112(5), 730-738.
- **World Food Programme. (2020).** Democratic Republic of Congo: Nutrition.
- **World Health Organization. (2019).** Integrated care protocols: a training guide **World Health Organization. (2017).** Nutrient profiling: Report of a WHO/IASO Technical Meeting.

Websites and Organizations :

- Academy of Nutrition and Dietetics (AND) - www.eatright.org
- European Society for Clinical Nutrition and Metabolism (ESPEN) - www.espen.orgWorld Health Organization (WHO) - www. who .int/nutrition/en/

PART 2: MENU PREPARATION AND THERAPEUTIC FOODS

INTRODUCTION

In the field of nutrition and health, the preparation of ready-to-use menus and therapeutic foods plays an important role. Whether for people suffering from chronic diseases, metabolic disorders, or those requiring a specific diet for medical reasons, the quality and appropriateness of the meals prepared are essential to promote well-being and healing.

This course aims to provide healthcare professionals, nutritionists and anyone interested in the subject with the knowledge they need to develop menus and foods adapted to the therapeutic needs of individuals. We will cover the basic principles of therapeutic nutrition, specific dietary requirements for different medical conditions, as well as menu preparation and management techniques. During the course, we will also explore the challenges and opportunities associated with the preparation of ready-to-use therapeutic foods, including ingredient quality, budgetary and logistical constraints, as well as regulatory and food safety aspects.

Combining theory and practice, this course aims to provide students with the necessary tools to create balanced and adapted menus, thus promoting better management of medical conditions through appropriate nutrition. The course objectives are:

1. Understand the basic principles of therapeutic nutrition.
2. Learn how to plan balanced menus that meet the specific nutritional needs of target populations.
3. Explore ready-to-use therapeutic food options and how to incorporate

them into menus.

4. Acquire practical skills in preparing and handling therapeutic foods.
5. Evaluate the effectiveness of menus and therapeutic foods in the management of specific medical conditions.

CHAPTER 10: INTRODUCTION TO THERAPEUTIC NUTRITION

Introduction

An introduction to therapeutic nutrition involves understanding how the food we eat can impact our physical and mental health. Unlike traditional nutrition, which focuses primarily on maintaining a balanced diet to prevent disease and promote general well-being, therapeutic nutrition concentrates on the specific use of food to treat or alleviate the symptoms of various medical conditions.

10.1 Key principles of therapeutic nutrition :

1. **Specific nutrients for specific conditions:** therapeutic nutrition recognizes that certain nutrients can have specific effects on certain diseases or conditions. For example, the use of certain vitamins, minerals, fatty acids or antioxidants may be beneficial in treating or preventing certain diseases.
2. **Personalization:** in contrast to a generic approach, therapeutic nutrition is often customized to the patient's individual needs, specific health conditions, food allergies and dietary preferences.
3. **Balance:** although therapeutic nutrition may involve specific adjustments to the diet to treat a particular disease, it always aims to maintain an overall nutritional balance. Nutritional deficiencies must be avoided while working to improve health.
4. **Multidisciplinary collaboration:** in practice, therapeutic nutrition often involves collaboration between different healthcare

professionals, such as nutritionists, physicians, dieticians and therapists, to develop effective nutritional plans for patients.

5. **Education and empowerment:** an important aspect of nutrition therapy is educating patients about food choices and the effects of these choices on their health. Empowering patients to make informed decisions about their diet is essential to promoting long-term health.
6. **Ongoing evaluation:** therapeutic nutrition plans must be evaluated regularly to ensure their effectiveness, and to make adjustments if necessary in response to changes in the patient's state of health.

In conclusion, therapeutic nutrition is a holistic approach to health that recognizes the crucial role of diet in the treatment and prevention of disease. By understanding how different foods and nutrients interact with the body, it is possible to design personalized nutritional plans that support long-term health and well-being.

10.2 Definitions and key concepts

Here are a few definitions and key concepts in nutrition therapy, with details and examples:

1. **Macronutrients:** macronutrients are the food components needed in large quantities to provide energy and support essential bodily functions. They include carbohydrates, proteins and lipids.

- For example, people with diabetes can benefit from precise management of their carbohydrate intake to control blood sugar levels.

2. **Micronutrients:** micronutrients are vitamins and minerals needed in small quantities to maintain optimal health and support specific bodily processes.

- Example: pregnant women may need folate supplements to prevent neural tube defects in the fetus.

3. **Antioxidants:** antioxidants are compounds found in foods that help protect cells against damage caused by free radicals, helping to prevent chronic disease and premature aging.

- For example, fruits and vegetables rich in vitamin C, such as oranges and red peppers, are important sources of antioxidants.

4. **Inflammation:** inflammation is a natural response of the immune system to aggression, but chronic inflammation can contribute to the development of many diseases, including cardiovascular disease, diabetes and autoimmune disorders. - Example: certain omega-3 fatty acids, found in oily fish such as salmon and sardines, have anti-inflammatory properties that can help reduce inflammation in the body.

5. **Glycemic index (GI):** the glycemic index is a measure of how quickly a food raises blood sugar levels after consumption. High-GI foods can cause a rapid rise in blood sugar levels, which can be problematic for people with diabetes or wishing to control their weight.

- Example: high-GI foods include candy, sodas and white flour baked goods, while non-starchy vegetables, legumes and whole grains tend to have a lower GI.

6. **Food intolerances:** food intolerances occur when the body has difficulty digesting certain foods, which can lead to uncomfortable digestive symptoms such as bloating, abdominal pain and diarrhea.

- Example: people with celiac disease are intolerant to gluten, a protein found in wheat, barley and rye, which can cause damage to their small intestine.

By understanding these key concepts, individuals can make informed dietary decisions to support their overall health and well-being, as well as to treat or alleviate the symptoms of certain medical conditions.

10.3 Development of nutritional plans for patients with various medical conditions

Developing nutritional plans for patients with different medical conditions requires a personalized approach to each specific case.

Some general guidelines for common medical conditions:

1. Diabetes and obesity:

Limit consumption of simple sugars and refined carbohydrates.

Encourage the consumption of dietary fibre, whole grains, fruits and vegetables. Control portions and spread meals throughout the day to maintain stable blood sugar levels.

Monitor carbohydrate intake and adjust insulin or hypoglycemic medication doses accordingly.

Favour lean proteins and healthy fats

Example 1: people with type 2 diabetes can benefit from a high-fiber diet, with low-glycemic carbohydrates, to avoid blood sugar spikes after meals.

Example 2: for people with obesity, a diet rich in vegetables, fruit, whole grains and lean proteins can promote weight loss and improve cardiovascular risk factors.

2. Hypertension :

Limit salt and sodium-rich foods.

Encourage consumption of potassium-rich foods, such as fruits and vegetables. Encourage magnesium-rich foods, especially green vegetables, nuts and seeds.

Reduce alcohol and caffeine consumption.

3. Hypercholesterolemia :

Limit saturated and trans fats, found in processed and fried foods. Favor unsaturated fats, such as those found in avocados, nuts, seeds and oily fish.

Encourage consumption of soluble fiber, found in fruits, vegetables, legumes and wholegrain cereals.

Incorporate foods rich in plant sterols, such as enriched margarines.

4. Heart disease :

Reduce consumption of saturated and trans fats.

Encourage consumption of fish, especially varieties rich in omega fatty acids.

Limit foods high in cholesterol, such as eggs and organ meats.

Favoring antioxidant-rich foods, such as colorful fruits and vegetables. Example: the Mediterranean diet, characterized by an abundance of fruits, vegetables, whole grains, olive oil and fish, is associated with a reduced risk of cardiovascular disease.

5. **Cancer:**

Adapt your diet to the type of cancer you have and the treatments you are undergoing.

Encourage consumption of foods rich in antioxidants and phytonutrients.

Ensure adequate protein intake to promote healing and recovery.

Monitor gastrointestinal symptoms and adapt diet accordingly.

6. **Renal insufficiency :**

Control protein intake, especially animal proteins.

Limit salt, potassium and phosphorus intake, depending on the stage of kidney disease.

Encourage consumption of low-potassium fruits and vegetables.

Monitor fluid intake and adjust according to degree of renal impairment.

In all cases, it's essential to work closely with a healthcare professional, such as a dietician or nutritionist, to develop a nutritional plan tailored to each patient's specific needs, and to ensure regular follow-up to adjust the plan according to progress and changes in the medical condition.

7. **Managing inflammatory diseases:** some foods may have anti-inflammatory properties that can help alleviate the symptoms of inflammatory diseases such as rheumatoid arthritis, Crohn's disease and ulcerative colitis ()[1] .

[1] *Dietary fibers, the natural prebiotics found in fruits, vegetables, legumes and whole*

Example: foods rich in omega-3 fatty acids, such as oily fish, nuts and seeds, can reduce inflammation and relieve joint pain in arthritis sufferers.

8. **Immune system support:** a diet rich in essential nutrients such as vitamins A, C, D, E, zinc and selenium can boost the immune system and help prevent infections.

For example, citrus fruits, berries, green leafy vegetables, nuts and seeds are all foods rich in vitamins and minerals that support immune function. By understanding how food choices can influence health and well-being, it becomes clear that nutrition plays a crucial role in the management and prevention of a wide range of medical conditions. By adopting a balanced diet tailored to their individual needs, individuals can improve their quality of life and reduce their risk of developing chronic health problems.

10.4 Basic principles of nutritional planning

Nutritional planning is based on several basic principles designed to ensure adequate nutrient intake to support health and well-being. Here are some of these principles, with details and illustrations:

1. **Nutritional balance:** a balanced diet includes a variety of foods from all food groups, including fruits, vegetables, whole grains, lean proteins and dairy or alternative products. The aim is to obtain a

grains, are particularly beneficial to the health of the intestinal microbiota by promoting the growth of beneficial bacteria.

Fermented foods, such as yogurt, kefir, sauerkraut and miso, contain natural probiotics that can help reseed the gut microbiota with beneficial bacteria.

range of essential nutrients to support bodily functions and prevent deficiencies.

-Illustration: a balanced meal might include grilled chicken (protein), brown rice (complex carbohydrates), steamed vegetables (fiber, vitamins and minerals) and a salad (varied nutrients).

2. **Variety:** eating a variety of foods ensures a diversified intake of nutrients, which contributes to overall health and the prevention of nutritional deficiencies. -Illustration: instead of eating the same vegetables every day, vary your choice by including vegetables of different colors, such as orange carrots, green spinach and red peppers.

3. **Moderation:** moderation means eating foods high in calories, saturated fats, added sugars and sodium sparingly, while favoring healthier food choices.

- Illustration: rather than eating a large slice of chocolate cake, opt for a small portion as an occasional treat and balance it with more nutritious food choices.

4. **Adequacy:** Adequacy means consuming appropriate amounts of food to meet individual energy and nutrient requirements, according to age, gender, level of physical activity and any specific health conditions.

- Illustration: the energy requirements of a top-level athlete will be higher than those of a sedentary person, so his or her diet will need to provide sufficient calories to support sporting performance.

5. **Fresh and unprocessed:** fresh, unprocessed foods are generally

richer in nutrients and lower in added sugars, saturated fats and sodium than processed foods.

- Illustration: choose fresh fruit rather than canned fruit, or wholegrain cereals rather than processed, sugary cereals, for optimum nutritional intake.

6. **Adequate hydration:** drinking enough water is essential to maintain hydration, support bodily functions and promote good digestion.

- Illustration: in addition to drinking water, you can also get hydration from beverages like unsweetened tea, herbal teas or water-rich fruits like melon and watermelon.

By applying these basic principles of nutritional planning to your daily diet, you can optimize your health and well-being by providing your body with the nutrients it needs to function efficiently.

CHAPTER 11: ASSESSING NUTRITIONAL REQUIREMENTS

Introduction

Assessing nutritional needs is a crucial process in individual diet planning. It involves determining a person's specific nutrient requirements based on various factors such as age, gender, physical activity level, health status, food allergies and health goals. This assessment then provides a basis for developing a personalized nutritional plan that meets the specific nutritional needs of each individual.

The primary objective of a nutritional needs assessment is to ensure adequate intake of essential nutrients to support growth, development and optimal functioning of body organs and systems, as well as to prevent nutritional deficiencies and associated health problems. An accurate assessment of nutritional needs can also help manage and prevent chronic diseases such as obesity, diabetes, cardiovascular disease and gastrointestinal disorders.

11.1 Steps in assessing nutritional needs

This nutritional needs assessment process usually involves several steps, including :

1. **Data collection:** this stage involves gathering information on lifestyle, eating habits, medical history, food allergies and other relevant factors that could influence the person's nutritional needs.

2. **Anthropometric assessment:** this involves measuring parameters

such as weight, height, waist circumference and body fat percentage, in order to assess body composition and identify any weight or nutritional problems.

3. **Subjective nutritional assessment:** this involves asking the person about their eating habits, food preferences, nutritional symptoms and appetite level, in order to assess their current nutritional status.
4. **Objective nutritional assessment:** this stage involves analysis of dietary intake using food diaries, food recalls or diet monitoring tools to assess macro- and micronutrient intake.
5. **Assessment of specific needs:** based on the data collected, specific needs in calories, macronutrients (carbohydrates, proteins, lipids) and micronutrients (vitamins, minerals, antioxidants) are calculated and adjusted according to individual health objectives.
6. **Drawing up a nutritional plan:** finally, on the basis of the nutritional needs assessment, a personalized food plan is developed, highlighting specific dietary recommendations to meet the person's nutritional needs, while taking into account their food preferences and individual constraints.

In conclusion, assessing nutritional needs is a fundamental step in the nutritional planning process, aimed at ensuring adequate nutrient intake to support individual health and well-being. By understanding the specific nutritional needs of each individual, it becomes possible to design personalized food plans that promote a healthy, balanced diet, while helping to achieve specific health goals.

11.2 Main medical conditions requiring nutritional intervention

There are many medical conditions for which nutritional intervention can play a crucial role in symptom management, treatment and prevention of complications. Here are some of the major medical conditions that often require nutritional intervention, with details and illustrations:

1. **Diabetes:** diabetes is a chronic disease characterized by high blood sugar levels. A balanced diet and management of carbohydrate intake are essential to control blood sugar levels in people with diabetes.

- Illustration: people with diabetes can benefit from a high-fiber diet, with low-glycemic carbohydrates such as vegetables, fruit, legumes and whole grains, to help maintain stable blood sugar levels.

2. **Cardiovascular disease:** cardiovascular disease, including high blood pressure, coronary heart disease and stroke, can be influenced by diet. A healthy diet can help reduce the risk of developing these diseases and improve heart health.

- Illustration: a diet rich in fruits, vegetables, whole grains, oily fish, nuts and seeds, while limiting consumption of saturated fats, sodium and added sugars, can help reduce the risk of cardiovascular disease.

3. **Obesity:** obesity is a major risk factor for many diseases, including diabetes, cardiovascular disease, metabolic disorders and certain types of cancer. A balanced diet and portion management can help achieve and maintain a healthy body weight.

- Illustration: to lose weight in a healthy way, it is recommended to follow a balanced diet including a variety of nutritious foods, controlling portions and limiting foods rich in empty calories.

4. **Inflammatory bowel disease (IBD):** Inflammatory bowel diseases, such as Crohn's disease and ulcerative colitis, can be influenced by diet. Some foods can trigger flare-ups or worsen symptoms, while others can bring relief.

- Illustration: for some people with IBD, a low-fiber diet may help reduce inflammation and gastrointestinal symptoms, while others may benefit from a diet rich in soluble fiber to promote intestinal health.

5. **Kidney disease:** chronic kidney disease can affect the balance of nutrients in the body, often requiring adjustments in diet to reduce the load on the kidneys and prevent complications.

- Illustration: people with kidney disease can be encouraged to limit their intake of sodium, potassium and phosphorus, while monitoring their protein intake to reduce renal burden.

In summary, nutritional intervention is often essential in the management of many medical conditions. By understanding how diet can influence the health and symptoms of these conditions, it is possible to develop personalized dietary plans that support overall health and improve patients' quality of life.

11.3 Assessment of the specific nutritional needs of target populations

Assessing the specific nutritional needs of target populations is essential to designing effective nutrition programs that meet the unique needs of each demographic group. Here are some examples of target populations and details of their specific nutritional needs:

1. **Children and infants :**
   - Children's nutritional requirements are higher per unit of body weight than those of adults, due to their rapid growth,
   - infants need an adequate intake of proteins, fats, carbohydrates, vitamins and minerals to support physical and cognitive development,
   - Exclusive breastfeeding is recommended for the first six months of life, as breast milk provides essential nutrients and strengthens the baby's immune system.
2. **Pregnant and breast-feeding women:**
   - Pregnant women have increased nutritional needs due to foetal growth and metabolic changes,
   - they need extra folic acid, iron, calcium and other nutrients to support the health of both mother and baby,
   - Breastfeeding women have increased nutritional requirements to produce quality breast milk and provide essential nutrients for their babies.
3. **Seniors :**
   - Elderly people often have different nutritional needs due to age-related physiological changes, such as reduced muscle mass and reduced nutrient absorption,
   - they may require higher intakes of protein, calcium, vitamin D and vitamin B12 to maintain muscle, bone and cognitive health,

- the elderly are often at greater risk of dehydration, so it's important to monitor their fluid intake.

4. **Athletes and sportsmen :**

- Athletes have increased nutritional requirements due to their intense physical activity and high energy demands,
- they require an adequate intake of carbohydrates for energy, proteins for muscle recovery, and electrolytes to maintain hydration and fluid balance,
- Macronutrient and micronutrient requirements may vary according to the type of physical activity, training intensity and individual goals.

5. **People with chronic diseases :**

- People with chronic illnesses such as diabetes, cardiovascular disease and kidney disease may have specific nutritional needs to manage their condition,
- they may require strict glycemic control, reduced sodium intake, increased fiber intake, or other dietary adjustments specific to their medical condition.

In conclusion, assessing the specific nutritional requirements of target populations is essential to designing nutrition programs tailored to their unique needs. By understanding the particular nutritional requirements of each demographic group, it is possible to promote healthy eating and support the health and well-being of these populations.

11.4 Use of nutritional references for menu planning

The use of nutritional references is crucial in menu planning, whether for restaurants, school canteens, healthcare facilities or even diet-conscious individuals. Here's how nutritional references are used, and a few illustrations to help you understand:

1. Identifying nutritional needs: nutritional references, such as the Dietary Reference Intakes (DRIs) or the Recommended Daily Allowances (RDAs), provide guidelines on the amount of nutrients needed to maintain health.

- Illustration: GDAs indicate that an average adult needs around 2,000 calories a day, with specific recommendations for macronutrients (carbohydrates, lipids, proteins) and micronutrients (vitamins, minerals).

2. Developing balanced menus: using nutritional references as a guide, menu planners can create balanced meals that meet the nutritional needs of customers or consumers.

- Illustration: a balanced lunch menu might include a green salad with mixed vegetables (providing fiber, vitamins and minerals), a fillet of grilled fish (source of lean protein and omega-3 fatty acids), brown rice (complex carbohydrates) and a portion of fresh fruit.

3. **Diversity and variety:** nutritional references encourage a diversified diet, providing a range of essential nutrients from different food sources. - Illustration: a varied menu might include vegetarian options such as beans and lentils (sources of plant protein and fiber), whole grains such as quinoa or barley (complex

carbohydrates), and fruits and vegetables of different colors for a variety of vitamins and minerals.

4. **Reducing health risks:** by taking into account nutritional recommendations, menu planners can help reduce the risk of chronic diseases such as obesity, diabetes, cardiovascular disease and certain forms of cancer.

- Illustration: by limiting the use of ingredients rich in saturated fats, added sugars and sodium, menus can help promote healthier eating and reduce the risk of chronic diseases associated with poor diet.

5. **Education and awareness:** by displaying nutritional information on menus, consumers are informed about the food choices they make, which can encourage them to opt for healthier options.

- Illustration: restaurants and school canteens often display calories, fats, carbohydrates and proteins on their menus, enabling customers to make more informed food choices based on their individual nutritional needs.

In short, the use of nutritional references in menu planning is essential to ensure that the meals served meet consumers' nutritional needs and help promote a healthy, balanced diet.

CHAPTER 12: PLANNING THERAPEUTIC MENUS

Introduction

Therapeutic menu planning is a specific approach to meal planning that aims to use food as a therapeutic tool to treat or alleviate the symptoms of various medical conditions. Unlike traditional menu planning, which typically focuses on taste, variety and satisfying food preferences, therapeutic menu planning focuses on providing specific foods that can help improve health and manage medical conditions. The main objective of therapeutic menu planning is to design meals that meet the specific nutritional needs of people with certain diseases or conditions, while taking into account dietary restrictions and medical recommendations. This may include adapting nutrient intake, modifying food texture, limiting certain ingredients or promoting health-promoting foods.

12.1 Key principles of therapeutic menu planning include:

1. **Personalization:** menus are adapted to each patient's individual needs, based on their state of health, food allergies, dietary preferences and therapeutic goals.
2. **Nutritional balance:** meals are designed to provide an appropriate balance of macronutrients (carbohydrates, proteins, lipids) and micronutrients (vitamins, minerals, antioxidants) to meet the specific nutritional needs of each patient.
3. **Portion control:** portions are controlled to help maintain a healthy

body weight and control risk factors associated with certain diseases, such as obesity, diabetes and cardiovascular disease.

4. **Education and empowerment:** patients are educated about food choices that support their health and well-being, and are encouraged to actively participate in planning their therapeutic meals.
5. **Interdisciplinary collaboration:** healthcare professionals, including nutritionists, physicians and dieticians, work together to develop effective therapeutic food plans tailored to each patient.

In conclusion, therapeutic menu planning is a holistic approach to nutrition that recognizes the important role of food in the treatment and management of disease. By designing meals tailored to the specific needs of each patient, it is possible to support the health and improve the quality of life of people with a variety of medical conditions.

12.2 Development of balanced menus for various medical conditions (diabetes, cardiovascular disease, malnutrition, etc.).

Developing balanced menus for different medical conditions requires a thorough understanding of the specific nutritional requirements associated with each condition. Here are some sample menus for different medical conditions, with details of the nutritional principles to be observed:

1. **Diabetes** :

Breakfast :

- Oat flakes with berries and nuts.

- Vegetable omelette.
- Wholemeal or whole-grain bread.
- Unsweetened tea or coffee.

Lunch :

- Grilled chicken salad with mixed greens.
- Quinoa or brown rice.
- A handful of nuts.
- Unsweetened water or herbal tea.

Dinner :

- Baked fish with grilled vegetables.
- Green salad with olive oil vinaigrette.
- Sweet potato.
- Unsweetened water or herbal tea.

2. Cardiovascular diseases :

Breakfast :

- Plain Greek yogurt with fresh fruit and chia seeds.
- Wholemeal rye bread.
- Natural fruit juice with no added sugar.

Lunch :

- Grilled salmon fillet with spinach sautéed in garlic.
- Quinoa or lentils.
- Tomato and cucumber salad with a light vinaigrette.
- Water or green tea.

Dinner :

- Skinless roast chicken with steamed broccoli.
- Baked potatoes.
- Endive salad with walnuts and olive oil vinaigrette.
- Unsweetened water or herbal tea.

3. Malnutrition :

Breakfast :

- Fruit and vegetable smoothie (banana, spinach, avocado, almond milk).
- Wholemeal bread with almond butter or protein-rich cheese spread.
- Milk or enriched vegetable alternative.

Lunch :

- Grilled chicken with green beans sautéed in garlic and lemon.
- Whole-grain rice or quinoa.
- Fruit compote with no added sugar.

Dinner :

- Vegetarian chili with kidney beans, vegetables and corn.
- Lentil salad with vegetables and herbs.
- Plain Greek yogurt with berries.

For all these conditions, it is important to follow certain general nutritional principles:

- limit simple sugars and processed foods,
- Favour fibre-rich foods such as fruits, vegetables and whole grains,

- include lean or vegetable protein sources,
- use healthy fats such as olive oil, avocados and nuts, - control portions to maintain a healthy weight and avoid overeating.

It is advisable to consult a healthcare professional or nutritionist to personalize these menus according to individual needs and dietary preferences.

12.3 Adapting menus to suit dietary restrictions and individual preferences

Adapting menus to suit dietary restrictions and individual preferences is essential to ensure a balanced diet tailored to each person. Here are some tips for adapting menus:

1. Food allergies :

- identify specific allergens and avoid them altogether on menus,
- replace problematic foods with safe alternatives,
- example: replace cow's milk with almond milk or soya milk for people allergic to lactose. **2 Food intolerances:**
- eliminate foods that are poorly tolerated or difficult to digest,
- opt for appropriate alternatives to avoid uncomfortable symptoms,
- example: using gluten-free pasta for people suffering from celiac disease or gluten intolerance. **3. Food preferences :**
- take into account individual tastes and culinary preferences,
- offer a variety of options to suit everyone's preferences,
- example: offer vegetarian or vegan options for those who prefer to avoid meat or animal products.

Here are some examples of menus adapted to suit dietary restrictions and individual preferences:

Menu 1 :

Breakfast :

- Fruit smoothie (banana, strawberries, spinach) with almond milk.
- Gluten-free bread toast with almond butter.

Lunch :

- Mediterranean salad with quinoa, grilled vegetables, olives and feta (or a vegan alternative).
- Lemon water.

Dinner :

- Chickpea curry with basmati rice.
- Steamed broccoli.
- Green salad with olive oil and balsamic vinegar vinaigrette.

Menu 2 :

Breakfast :

- oat flakes cooked in coconut milk with berries and chia seeds.
- Mango and coconut smoothie®.

Lunch :

- vegetarian wrap® with grilled vegetables, avocado and salsa.
- sweet potato chips.
- plain soy yogurt.

Dinner :

- grilled salmon with dill sauce.
- roasted potatoes with garlic and rosemary.
- asparagus sautéed in olive oil.

By adapting menus to suit dietary restrictions and individual preferences, we can ensure a healthy, satisfying diet for everyone.

12.4 Ingredient substitution techniques to meet specific nutritional needs

Ingredient substitution techniques are useful for meeting specific nutritional requirements while taking into account dietary restrictions, individual preferences or special diets. Here are some common techniques with examples of substitute ingredients:

1. Dairy product substitution:

- For people who are lactose intolerant or following a vegan diet:
- Soy milk, almond milk, coconut milk or oat milk to replace cow's milk.
- Soy, almond or coconut yoghurt.
- Vegetable cheese made with cashew nuts or nutritional yeast.

2. Animal protein substitution :

- For vegetarian or vegan diets:
- Tofu, tempeh, seitan or edamame to replace meat.
- Lentils, beans, chickpeas and other legumes as sources of protein.
- Quinoa, brown rice or other protein-rich wholegrain cereals.

3. Refined carbohydrate substitution :

- To encourage more nutritious choices:
- Almond flour, coconut flour or chickpea flour to replace white flour.
- Wholegrain rice, quinoa, millet or spelt instead of white rice.
- Whole-wheat pasta, chickpea pasta or lentil pasta instead of traditional pasta.

4. Saturated fat substitution :

- For more heart-healthy options:
- Olive oil, avocado oil or non-hydrogenated coconut oil instead of butter or margarine.
- Crushed avocado or nut purée as a substitute for mayonnaise in sandwiches or salads.
- Nuts, chia seeds or flax seeds to enrich dishes with omega-3 fatty acids.

5. Sweetener substitution :

- To reduce your intake of added sugar:
- Stevia, pure maple syrup or raw honey instead of white sugar.
- Fruit puree (mashed banana, unsweetened applesauce) to sweeten recipes without adding refined sugar.
- Crushed dates or vanilla extract to add sweetness to desserts.

6. Substitution of common allergens :

- For people allergic to certain foods:
- Buckwheat flour, rice flour or corn flour to replace wheat flour.

- Almond milk, rice milk or hemp milk for people allergic to cow's milk.
- Seed butter (sunflower butter, sesame butter) to replace peanut butter for people allergic to peanuts.

By using these ingredient substitution techniques, it is possible to create balanced meals tailored to each individual's specific nutritional needs, while taking into account individual preferences and dietary restrictions.

CHAPTER 13: SELECTION AND INTEGRATION OF THERAPEUTIC FOODS

Introduction

Food plays a crucial role in promoting health and treating disease. Many foods possess therapeutic properties, offering specific health benefits and helping to prevent or treat certain medical conditions. The judicious selection and integration of these therapeutic foods into the daily diet can be an essential aspect of overall health management.

The use of therapeutic foods is based on a thorough understanding of the bioactive compounds present in foods, such as antioxidants, vitamins, minerals, essential fatty acids, dietary fiber and other beneficial nutrients. These compounds can have anti-inflammatory, antioxidant and antimicrobial effects, as well as regulating metabolism and boosting the immune system.

In this series on selecting and integrating therapeutic foods, we'll explore various medical conditions such as diabetes, cardiovascular disease, gastrointestinal disorders, inflammatory conditions, among others. We'll look at the specific foods recommended for each condition, as well as the mechanisms by which these foods can exert their beneficial effects.

We'll also cover practical strategies for incorporating these therapeutic foods into balanced, delicious meals, as well as tips for ensuring that the overall diet remains tailored to individual nutritional needs and food preferences.

The aim of this series is to provide an in-depth understanding of therapeutic foods and practical advice on how to incorporate them into a daily diet, helping to optimize everyone's health and well-being.

13.1 Types of ready-to-use therapeutic foods available on the market

There is a growing variety of ready-to-use therapeutic foods on the market, designed to meet specific health needs. These foods are often enriched with beneficial nutrients or formulated to offer health benefits. Here are some common types of therapeutic foods available on the market, with examples:

1. Energy and nutrition bars :

- These bars are often enriched with protein, fiber, vitamins and minerals to provide a nutritious and convenient snack.
- Examples: Protein bars, fruit and nut bars enriched with vitamins and minerals.

2. Functional drinks :

- Functional beverages are formulated to offer specific health benefits, such as energy, digestion or joint health.
- Examples: Protein drinks, probiotic drinks for intestinal health, energy drinks enriched with B vitamins.

3. Fermented foods :

- These foods contain probiotics that are beneficial to intestinal health and can help boost the immune system.
- Examples: probiotic yoghurts, kefir, lacto-fermented sauerkraut, kimchi.

4. **Meal replacements :**

- These products are designed to provide complete nutritional balance in a convenient format, often used as meal replacements for weight loss or blood sugar management.
- Examples: Nutritional milkshakes, protein soups, meal replacements rich in fibre and vitamins.

5. **Foods rich in omega-3 :**

- Foods enriched with omega-3 fatty acids are beneficial for heart health, brain function and reducing inflammation.
- Examples: Omega-3-enriched eggs, DHA-enriched almond milk, cold-pressed linseed oil.

6. **Healthy snacks :**

- These snacks are formulated to be nutrient-rich yet low in calories and added sugars.
- Examples: Whole-grain crackers, vegetable chips, mixed nuts, dried fruit with no added sugar.

7. **Fortified foods :**

- Some foods are enriched with vitamins, minerals or other specific nutrients to fill nutritional gaps.
- Examples: Cereals enriched with iron and folic acid, milk enriched with calcium and vitamin D, bread enriched with fiber.

13.2. For children suffering from acute malnutrition,

It's essential to provide nutrient-rich therapeutic foods to help them recover and get back on the road to health. Here are some examples of therapeutic foods suitable for children in this situation:

1. Ready-to-use nutritional paste (RUTF - Ready-to-Use Therapeutic Food): - This paste is specially formulated to be highly nutritious and energetic, providing a large quantity of calories, proteins, vitamins and minerals in a small quantity of volume;

- it is often used to treat severe malnutrition in children, as it is easy to administer and requires no preparation, e.g. Plumpy'Nut, Nutributter.

2. Enriched therapeutic milk :

- Therapeutic milk formulas are available for malnourished children, providing a source of high-quality protein and essential vitamins and minerals;
- These milks can be used to supplement children's diets and help them recover from malnutrition,
- example: nutrient-enriched therapeutic milk (F75 and F100 therapeutic milks).

3. Therapeutic cereal-based porridge:

- special porridges enriched with protein, iron, zinc and other nutrients are designed for children suffering from malnutrition;
- they provide an easy-to-digest source of energy and nutrients for children recovering from illness,
- example: porridge based on enriched cereal flours.

4. Vitamin and mineral supplements:

- vitamin and mineral supplements can be used to make up for nutritional deficiencies in malnourished children;

- they are often administered in the form of drops or tablets dispersible in water, e.g. vitamin A, C, D, iron and zinc supplements.

5. Enriched convenience foods :

- some ready-to-eat foods are enriched with essential nutrients and can be included in the diet of malnourished children to boost their nutritional intake;
- For example: yoghurts enriched with calcium and vitamins, cookies enriched with iron and B vitamins.

It is important to stress that the treatment of acute malnutrition in children often requires a comprehensive medical and nutritional approach, and these therapeutic foods must be administered under the supervision of a qualified health professional. In addition, it is essential to promote exclusive breastfeeding for infants and provide ongoing nutritional support to help prevent relapse of malnutrition.

13.3 Selection criteria for therapeutic foods based on nutritional requirements and patient preferences

When selecting therapeutic foods to meet patients' nutritional needs and preferences, it's important to consider a number of criteria to ensure an effective and appropriate diet. Here are some criteria to consider:

1. Nutritional composition :

- Choose foods rich in the essential nutrients required to meet the patient's specific needs. This may include proteins, complex carbohydrates, healthy fats, vitamins and minerals.

- Example: Select iron-rich foods for patients with anemia, calcium-rich foods for patients with osteoporosis.

2. Easy to digest :

- Choose foods that are easy to digest, especially if the patient has gastrointestinal problems or difficulty eating.
- Example: Choose cooked rather than raw foods to aid digestion.

3. Food preferences :

- Take into account the patient's food likes and dislikes to ensure that they consume the selected foods.
- Example: Offer vegetarian alternatives for patients who prefer to avoid meat, or sweet foods for patients with a sweet tooth.

4. Food restrictions and allergies :

- Ensure that the foods selected do not contain any known allergens or are not contraindicated due to the patient's specific dietary restrictions.
- Example: Avoid gluten-containing foods for celiac patients, or sodium-rich foods for hypertensive patients.

5. Texture and presentation :

- Select foods adapted to the patient's preferred texture, taking into account their ability to chew and swallow.
- Example: Offer chopped or puréed food for patients with swallowing difficulties.

6. Availability and cost :

- Choose foods that are easily accessible and affordable for patients, depending on their financial resources and geographical location.

- Example: Opt for local and seasonal foods, which are often less expensive and easier to find.

By taking these criteria into account when selecting therapeutic foods, it is possible to design food plans tailored to the specific nutritional needs and individual preferences of each patient. It is also advisable to consult a healthcare professional or nutritionist for personalized advice based on the patient's medical situation and needs.

13.4 Integrating therapeutic foods into menus for optimize their efficiency

The effective integration of therapeutic foods into menus involves incorporating them in a balanced and appropriate way, while taking into account the patient's specific nutritional needs. Here are some details on how to optimize the effectiveness of therapeutic foods in menus:

1. Identifying nutritional needs :

- Before incorporating therapeutic foods into a menu, it's essential to understand the patient's specific nutritional needs based on their medical condition, food preferences and restrictions.

2. Selection of relevant therapeutic foods :

- Choose therapeutic foods that meet the patient's identified nutritional needs. Select foods rich in specific nutrients beneficial to the patient's health.

3. **Nutritional balance :**

- Make sure meals contain a balanced combination of proteins, carbohydrates, fats, vitamins and minerals to meet the patient's overall nutritional needs.

4. **Variety and diversity :**

- Incorporate a variety of therapeutic foods into your menus to ensure a complete nutritional intake and to avoid dietary monotony.
- Experiment with different types of food to offer varied and interesting options.

5. **Incorporation into familiar dishes:**

- Integrate therapeutic foods into dishes that are familiar and enjoyed by the patient, to improve food acceptance and enjoyment.
- Modify traditional recipes to include therapeutic ingredients without compromising taste or texture.

6. **Attractive presentation:**

- Take care with the presentation of your dishes, using appealing techniques to stimulate the appetite and make meals more enjoyable.
- Play with colors, textures and garnishes to create visually appealing meals.

7. **Follow-up and adjustment :**

- Carefully monitor the patient's response to the inclusion of therapeutic foods in his or her diet.
- Adapt menus to the patient's reactions, changes in medical condition and food preferences.

8. Education and support :

- Provide information and advice to patients on the benefits of therapeutic foods and how to integrate them optimally into their daily diet.

- Offer ongoing support to help patients maintain a healthy diet adapted to their needs.

By carefully and systematically integrating therapeutic foods into menus, it is possible to optimize their effectiveness in improving patient health and well-being. It is advisable to work in collaboration with a healthcare professional or nutritionist to design personalized menus based on each patient's specific needs.

CHAPTER 14: PREPARATION AND HANDLING OF THERAPEUTIC FOODS

Introduction

When it comes to preparing and handling therapeutic foods, a careful and precise approach is essential to ensure their efficacy and safety. Therapeutic foods are often specifically formulated to meet particular nutritional needs, and their preparation can play a crucial role in their ability to deliver the nutrients needed to improve individual health and well-being.

In this series on the preparation and handling of therapeutic foods, we'll explore various aspects of this process, focusing on good practices and important considerations. We'll cover topics such as ingredient selection, preparation techniques, food safety, proper storage and presentation of therapeutic foods.

The aim of this series is to provide healthcare professionals, nutritionists, chefs and anyone involved in the preparation and supply of therapeutic foods with the knowledge and skills they need to guarantee the quality and efficacy of these foods as part of a therapeutic diet.

By understanding the fundamentals of therapeutic food preparation and handling, it is possible to optimize their contribution to the health and well-being of individuals, ensuring that they receive the nutrients they need to support their medical treatment and promote recovery.

14.1 Safe and hygienic preparation techniques for therapeutic foods

The safe and hygienic preparation of therapeutic foods is essential to ensure patient food safety and the preservation of the nutritional value of the food. Here are some techniques to follow, with details and examples:

1. **Hand washing :**

- wash hands thoroughly with soap and water before handling food. - example: before preparing a therapeutic porridge for a malnourished child, be sure to wash your hands for at least 20 seconds.

2. **Cleaning work surfaces :**

- Regularly clean and disinfect work surfaces, cutting boards and kitchen utensils to prevent cross-contamination.
- Example: Use a disinfectant solution to clean kitchen counters before preparing therapeutic foods.

3. **Use fresh, clean ingredients:**

- Use fresh, high-quality ingredients, making sure they are not contaminated by mold, parasites or bacteria.
- Example: Choose fruits and vegetables with no blemishes or signs of spoilage to make nutrient-rich therapeutic smoothies.

4. **Proper cooking :**

- Cook food at temperatures high enough to eliminate bacteria and ensure food safety.
- Example: Be sure to cook meats, eggs and dairy products to safe

internal temperatures recommended by health authorities.

5. Rapid cooling :

- Cool cooked food quickly to prevent the growth of pathogenic bacteria. - Example: Place hot food in a refrigerator or freezer immediately after cooking to cool it quickly.

6. Allergen handling :

- Avoid cross-contamination with known allergens by using clean utensils and separating allergenic from non-allergenic foods.
- Example: Use different knives and cutting boards for allergenic and non-allergenic foods.

7. Suitable storage :

- Store therapeutic foods in airtight containers, correctly labeled to preserve freshness and safety.
- Example: Store therapeutic porridges in individual containers in the fridge or freezer for later use.

8. Safety during service :

- Serve therapeutic foods at safe temperatures and ensure that they do not remain at room temperature for long periods.
- Example: Keep hot food in heated containers and cold food on ice during service events.

By following these safe and hygienic preparation techniques, it is possible to minimize the risk of food contamination and provide high-quality therapeutic foods that benefit patient health.

14.2 Proper storage and handling of ready-to-use therapeutic foods

Proper storage and handling of ready-to-use therapeutic foods is essential to ensure their efficacy, safety and nutritional quality. Here are some details and examples of how to store and handle these foods correctly:

1. Secure storage :

- Store therapeutic foods in a cool, dry place away from direct sunlight to preserve their freshness and quality.
- Make sure the storage area is clean and free of contaminants.

2. Monitoring best-before dates :

- Regularly check the expiration dates of therapeutic foods and use them before they expire to guarantee their safety and efficacy.
- Follow the manufacturer's instructions regarding shelf life after opening.

3. Protection against contamination :

- Store therapeutic foods in airtight containers or original packaging to avoid contamination by bacteria, mold or parasites. - Avoid storing food near chemicals, cleaning products or other potentially harmful substances.

4. Safe handling:

- When handling ready-to-use therapeutic foods, be sure to wash your hands thoroughly with soap and water before and after contact.
- Use clean, disinfected utensils for picking and handling food to

minimize the risk of contamination.

5. **Storage temperature :**

- Follow the manufacturer's recommendations on storage temperature for ready-to-use therapeutic foods.
- Keep refrigerated or frozen foods at the right temperature to prevent the growth of pathogenic bacteria.

6. **Clear labelling :**

- Properly label ready-to-use therapeutic foods with the necessary information, including opening date, expiration date and storage instructions.
- Make sure labels are clear and easy to read for easy identification and food management.

Examples:

- Ready-to-use nutritional pastes such as Plumpy'Nut should be stored in their original packaging, at room temperature, in a dry place and out of direct sunlight.
- Ready-to-use nutritional drinks should be kept refrigerated after opening, and consumed within the time recommended by the manufacturer to maintain freshness and safety.

By following these good storage and handling practices, it is possible to guarantee the quality, safety and efficacy of ready-to-use therapeutic foods, helping to improve the health and well-being of patients.

14.3 Special considerations for the preparation of therapeutic

foods for vulnerable populations (children, the elderly, etc.)

When preparing therapeutic foods for vulnerable populations such as children, the elderly or people with chronic diseases, it's important to take into account a number of special considerations to ensure their safety, efficacy and acceptability. Here are some details and examples of these considerations:

1. **Suitable texture :**

- For young children, the elderly or individuals with swallowing problems, it is often necessary to adapt the texture of therapeutic foods to make them easy to eat and digest.
- Example: Prepare smooth purées or soft foods for small children or elderly people with chewing difficulties.

2. **Portion size :**

- Take into account the specific calorie and nutrient requirements of each demographic group and adjust portion sizes accordingly.
- Example: Offer smaller but more frequent portions for children or the elderly with limited appetites.

3. **Variety of flavours :**

- Offer a variety of flavors and textures to stimulate appetite and increase acceptability of therapeutic foods.
- Example: Prepare fruit smoothies with different flavor combinations for children or the elderly.

4. **Familiar foods :**

- Use foods that are familiar and appreciated by the target

population to promote acceptability and encourage consumption.

- Example: Prepare soups or porridges based on traditional foods familiar to the elderly.

5. **Attractive presentation:**

- Make therapeutic foods visually appealing and appetizing, especially for children and the elderly.

- Example: Use playful shapes and bright colors for children's foods.

6. **Suitable consistency and temperature:**

- Ensure that therapeutic foods are served at the right temperature, neither too hot nor too cold, to avoid the risk of burns or digestive upsets.

- Example: Serve mashed potatoes hot, but not scalding hot, for the elderly or young children.

7. **Specific nutritional considerations :**

- Adapt therapeutic food recipes to meet the specific nutritional needs of each demographic group, taking into account calcium, iron, vitamin requirements, etc.

- Example: Enrich therapeutic foods for the elderly by adding sources of calcium to maintain bone health.

By taking these special considerations into account when preparing therapeutic foods for vulnerable populations, it is possible to ensure their efficacy, safety and acceptability, thereby helping to improve the health and well-being of these demographic groups.

CHAPTER 15: EVALUATING THE EFFECTIVENESS OF MENUS AND THERAPEUTIC FOODS

Introduction

Evaluating the effectiveness of menus and therapeutic foods is a crucial step in the management of therapeutic diets. It ensures that individuals' specific nutritional needs are met, that health goals are achieved, and that dietary interventions are appropriate and effective. In this series on evaluating the effectiveness of therapeutic menus and foods, we will explore various aspects of this evaluation, focusing on the methods, tools and indicators used to assess the appropriateness, effectiveness and impact of nutritional interventions.

We'll cover topics such as assessing nutritional intake, monitoring health parameters, evaluating patient satisfaction, and using clinical data to evaluate long-term outcomes. In addition, we will examine the challenges and special considerations involved in evaluating menus and therapeutic foods for different demographic groups, including children, the elderly and people with chronic diseases.

The aim of this series is to provide healthcare professionals, nutritionists, dieticians and other practitioners involved in prescribing and managing therapeutic diets with the knowledge and skills to critically and effectively evaluate the impact of nutritional interventions on individual health and well-being.

By understanding how to evaluate the effectiveness of menus and therapeutic foods, it's possible to optimize patients' nutritional management, identify necessary adjustments and provide ongoing support to promote positive health outcomes.

15.1 Monitoring patients' nutritional progress

Monitoring patients' nutritional progress is essential for evaluating the effectiveness of nutritional interventions, adjusting treatment plans and promoting positive health outcomes. Here are some details and examples of methods commonly used to monitor patients' nutritional progress:

1. **Assessment of food intake :**

- Use food diaries, food reminders or food frequency questionnaires to assess patients' daily nutritional intake.

- Example: Ask patients to keep a detailed food diary for a few days to record everything they eat, then analyze the data to assess their calorie, macronutrient and micronutrient intake.

2. **Body composition monitoring :**

- Regularly measure patients' body composition, including weight, height, waist circumference, fat mass and lean mass.

- Example: Use techniques such as regular weighing, waist circumference measurement and bio-impedance body composition analysis to track changes in weight and body composition over time.

3. **Analysis of biometric parameters :**

- Monitor patients' biometric parameters, such as blood glucose, cholesterol, blood pressure and blood lipid levels, to assess their metabolic and cardiovascular health.

- Example: Perform regular blood tests to monitor levels of glucose, glycated hemoglobin, lipids and other markers of metabolic health in diabetic patients.

4. **Assessment of symptoms :**

- Ask patients about nutritional symptoms such as fatigue, nausea, gastrointestinal disorders, etc., to assess the impact of their diet on their general well-being.

- Example: Use standardized nutrition-related quality of life questionnaires to assess the symptoms and well-being of patients with gastrointestinal diseases.

5. **Monitoring growth and development :**

- For children, monitor growth and physical, cognitive and psychosocial development to assess the impact of their diet on their overall health.

- Example: Use growth charts to monitor weight, height and motor development in infants and young children.

6. **Assessing patient satisfaction :**

- Gather patients' comments and impressions of their diet and nutritional experience to assess their satisfaction and adherence to dietary recommendations.

- Example: Administer patient satisfaction surveys to assess satisfaction with the proposed diet and identify potential areas for improvement.

By combining these different monitoring methods, it is possible to obtain a complete picture of patients' nutritional progress, and identify the adjustments needed to optimize their health and well-being. It is advisable to tailor monitoring to each patient's individual needs, and to work closely with a multidisciplinary healthcare team to ensure effective nutritional management.

15.2 Assessing patient and provider satisfaction

Assessing patient and provider satisfaction is essential to understanding the effectiveness of nutritional interventions, the patient experience and the overall impact of healthcare. Here are some details and examples of how to assess patient and provider satisfaction:

1. Patient satisfaction questionnaires:

- Administer structured questionnaires to patients to gather their opinions, concerns and suggestions regarding the nutrition services and care they have received.

- Example: a post-consultation satisfaction questionnaire where patients rate the quality of the information provided, the friendliness of the staff and their overall satisfaction with the nutrition consultation experience.

2. Individual interviews :

- Conduct one-on-one interviews with patients to learn more about their experience, understand their needs and expectations, and gather qualitative feedback.

- Example: A structured interview with a patient to discuss his perceptions of the relevance of dietary recommendations and how they have been implemented in his daily life. **3. Focus groups:**

- Organize focus groups with patients to explore specific themes, share similar experiences and encourage open communication.

- Example: a focus group with diabetic patients to discuss the challenges they face in managing their diet and to share strategies for success.

4. **Evaluation of complaints and comments :**

- Monitor and analyze patient complaints, comments and suggestions to identify areas for improvement and address concerns.

- Example: tracking patient comments left on social networking platforms, satisfaction surveys or feedback forms in healthcare facilities.

5. **Assessing provider satisfaction :**

- Gather impressions and opinions from care providers on the quality of nutrition services, interprofessional collaboration and their overall satisfaction with care delivery.

- Example: an anonymous survey of doctors, nurses and other healthcare professionals to assess their perception of the effectiveness of nutrition services in patient management.

6. **Analysis of operational data :**

- Analyze operational data such as waiting times, missed appointment rates and treatment times to assess the effectiveness of nutrition services from the patient's point of view.

- Example: tracking the average waiting time for an appointment with a dietician and comparing it with the time targets set by the healthcare facility.

By using these methods to assess patient and provider satisfaction, valuable information can be gathered to improve the delivery of nutrition services, enhance patient engagement and improve overall health outcomes. It is recommended that these assessments be implemented on a regular and ongoing basis to ensure continuous improvement in the quality of care.

15.3 Readjustment of menus and therapeutic foods according to results obtained

Adjusting menus and therapeutic foods according to the results obtained is an essential step in optimizing the effectiveness of nutritional interventions and meeting patients' changing needs. Here are a few details and examples of how to do this:

1. **Analysis of initial results :**

- Evaluate the results of previous nutritional interventions by comparing initial data with current data, such as body composition, biometric parameters, eating habits and symptoms.

2. **Identifying emerging needs :**

- Identify new nutritional needs or emerging health problems in patients, taking into account changes in medical conditions, treatment goals and individual preferences.

3. **Revision of nutritional targets :**

- Revise nutritional targets based on results obtained and needs identified, adjusting calorie intakes, specific nutrients and other dietary components according to individual patient needs.

- Example: Increase protein intake for a patient recovering from surgery or injury, or reduce sodium intake for a hypertensive patient.

4. **Menu adaptation :**

- Modify menus to better meet identified nutritional needs, by introducing new foods, adjusting portions and modifying preparation methods according to patients' preferences and dietary restrictions.

- Example: Include more iron sources in meals for a patient with anemia, or offer gluten-free options for a patient with celiac disease.

5. **Continuous monitoring and surveillance :**

- Carefully monitor patients' progress after dietary adjustments to assess their response and adherence to the new dietary plans.

- Example: Conduct regular follow-up visits to monitor changes in weight, body composition and biometric parameters, as well as to gather feedback from patients on their new eating habits.

6. **Interprofessional collaboration :**

- Collaborate with other healthcare professionals, such as doctors, nurses and therapists, to share information on patient progress and adjust treatment plans holistically.

- Example: Discuss nutritional results with the care team to determine whether adjustments in other areas of treatment are needed to support nutritional goals.

By regularly readjusting menus and therapeutic foods based on results achieved, it is possible to optimize the effectiveness of nutritional interventions, meet patients' changing needs and promote positive long-term health outcomes. It is recommended that dietary plans continue to be monitored and adjusted as patients' medical conditions and treatment goals evolve.

CHAPTER 16: CHALLENGES AND SOLUTIONS IN PREPARING MENUS AND THERAPEUTIC FOODS

Introduction

Preparing menus and therapeutic foods is a complex task that can face a variety of challenges. These challenges can include strict nutritional constraints, individual dietary preferences, budgetary restrictions and logistical constraints. Each challenge requires a thoughtful approach and tailored solutions to ensure that patients' nutritional needs are met safely and effectively. In this chapter on challenges and solutions in menu and therapeutic food preparation, we'll look in detail at common obstacles encountered by nutrition and healthcare professionals, as well as practical strategies for overcoming them. We'll look at the challenges of managing nutritional constraints, satisfying patients' dietary preferences, managing limited resources and the logistical challenges associated with preparing and distributing therapeutic foods.

The aim of this series is to provide healthcare professionals, nutritionists, dieticians and other practitioners involved in the preparation of menus and therapeutic foods with the knowledge and tools they need to effectively meet these challenges.

By understanding potential obstacles and learning how to implement practical solutions, it is possible to optimize the quality of nutritional care and improve patient health outcomes.

In this chapter, we'll explore various aspects of the challenges and solutions involved in preparing menus and therapeutic foods, highlighting concrete examples and best practices for meeting these challenges effectively and efficiently.

16.1 Logistical and financial challenges involved in preparing and supplying therapeutic foods

Logistical and financial challenges related to the preparation and supply of therapeutic foods can present significant obstacles to the provision of effective nutritional care. Here are some details and examples of these challenges, as well as potential solutions

1. Storage and distribution logistics :

- Challenge: therapeutic foods often require specific storage and handling conditions to guarantee their efficacy and safety. Managing these logistical requirements can be complex, particularly in healthcare establishments or in environments with limited resources.
- Solution: implement efficient inventory management systems, including appropriate receiving, storage and distribution protocols. Using technologies such as barcode tracking or computerized inventory management can also help optimize processes.
- Example: in healthcare establishments, create dedicated storage areas with controlled temperature and humidity conditions for sensitive therapeutic foods.

2. High cost of therapeutic foods:

- Challenge: special therapeutic foods can be expensive, which can represent a financial challenge for individuals, families or healthcare institutions, especially when large quantities are required over a long period.

- Solution: look for suppliers offering competitive prices and bulk purchasing options. Explore possibilities for reimbursement by health insurance programs or governments, as well as subsidies or support programs available to low-income people.
- Example: negotiate agreements with suppliers to obtain discounted rates on therapeutic foods by buying in large quantities or establishing partnerships with charitable organizations.

3. Limited availability of specific foods :

- Challenge: some therapeutic foods can be difficult to find or obtain, especially in remote areas or developing countries where access to specialized food products is limited.
- Solution: explore local alternatives or substitutions for hard-to-find foods. Partner with local suppliers or farmers to obtain specific products, or consider distribution or transportation programs for remote areas.
- Example: use nutrient-rich local foods to replace imported therapeutic foods, for example by using local legumes and cereals as sources of protein and complex carbohydrates.

By overcoming these logistical and financial challenges with creative solutions and strategic approaches, it is possible to ensure an effective and efficient supply of therapeutic foods, thereby helping to improve the health and well-being of patients.

16.2 Solutions to overcome obstacles to integrating therapeutic foods into menus

Integrating therapeutic foods into menus can face a variety of obstacles, including nutritional constraints, individual food preferences and logistical limitations. Here are some solutions for overcoming these obstacles, with details and examples:

1. Collaboration with nutritionists and dieticians:

- Solution: work closely with nutrition professionals to develop balanced menus adapted to patients' specific nutritional needs. - Example: a nutritionist can help design menus for diabetic patients, taking into account their carbohydrate intake, glycemic index and meal distribution throughout the day.

2. Education of chefs and kitchen staff :

- Solution: train kitchen staff in the preparation of therapeutic foods, focusing on healthy cooking techniques and appropriate ingredient substitutions.
- Example: organize training sessions where chefs learn how to prepare low-sodium meals for hypertensive patients, or gluten-free alternatives for celiac patients.

3. Diversification of food options :

- Solution: offer a variety of therapeutic foods to meet patients' different nutritional needs and dietary preferences.
- Example: propose vegan alternatives or plant-based protein options for patients preferring a plant-based diet or for those with dietary

restrictions of animal origin.

4. Gradual integration into existing menus:

- Solution: gradually introduce therapeutic foods into existing menus, combining them with familiar dishes to make the transition smoother.
- Example: Add fiber-rich vegetables and whole grains to traditional dishes like soups, stews or salads to boost their nutritional value.

5. Regular assessment of patient satisfaction:

- Solution: gather patient feedback on therapeutic meals to assess their acceptability and satisfaction, and make adjustments based on their feedback.
- Example: administer regular satisfaction surveys where patients can give their opinion on menus and offer suggestions for improvement.

By implementing these solutions and adopting a collaborative, patient-focused approach, it is possible to overcome the obstacles to integrating therapeutic foods into menus, thus guaranteeing a diet that is adapted and beneficial to patients' health.

16.3 The role of healthcare professionals and community workers in promoting nutrition therapy

Healthcare professionals and community stakeholders play a crucial role in promoting therapeutic nutrition by providing information, advice and support to individuals to optimize their nutritional health. Here are some details and examples of their role:

1. Education and awareness :

- Healthcare professionals and community workers can raise awareness of the benefits of a healthy, balanced diet, as well as the importance of therapeutic nutrition in the management of chronic diseases and medical conditions.

- Example: organize nutrition education sessions in schools, health centers or community centers to teach individuals the principles of a balanced diet and strategies for improving their nutritional health.

2. **Nutritional assessment and prescription :**

- Healthcare professionals, such as doctors, nutritionists and dieticians, can assess patients' individual nutritional needs and prescribe therapeutic diets tailored to their specific medical conditions.

- Example: a dietician prescribes a low-sodium, high-potassium diet for a hypertensive patient to reduce blood pressure and prevent cardiovascular complications. **3. Advice and support :**

- Provide personalized advice and support to individuals to help them implement positive dietary changes and maintain healthy eating habits over the long term.

- Example: a nurse provides advice on meal planning and strategies for managing food cravings in a diabetic patient to improve glycemic control.

4. **Promoting access to therapeutic foods :**

- Community stakeholders can play a role in promoting access to therapeutic foods by working with local suppliers, government organizations and charities to facilitate the distribution of these foods to individuals in need.

- Example: a community organization works with local food banks to include therapeutic foods in food baskets distributed to low-income families.

5. Education and support for caregivers :

- Provide information and resources to caregivers and family members to help them effectively support individuals on therapeutic diets.
- Example: organize training workshops for family caregivers on preparing meals adapted to the specific nutritional needs of the elderly or people with chronic illnesses.

By working together, healthcare professionals and community stakeholders can play a central role in promoting therapeutic nutrition, helping individuals achieve their nutritional health goals and improving overall health outcomes in the community.

CHAPTER 17: CASE STUDIES AND PRACTICAL APPLICATIONS

Introduction

The introduction of case studies and practical applications in the field of therapeutic nutrition offers a valuable opportunity to apply theoretical knowledge to real-life situations and understand how nutrition principles are implemented in clinical practice. In this series, we will explore different case studies and practical applications covering a wide range of medical conditions, specific nutritional needs and healthcare settings.

The aim of these case studies is to provide concrete examples of how healthcare professionals can assess, plan and implement effective nutritional interventions to meet individual patient needs. Each case study will be accompanied by a detailed analysis, highlighting clinical considerations, treatment decisions and outcomes achieved.

The hands-on applications will enable healthcare professionals to gain a practical understanding of nutritional concepts and learn how to adapt nutritional recommendations to specific patient needs. The applications will also provide practical advice on meal planning, preparing therapeutic foods and managing nutritional challenges encountered in clinical practice.

By exploring these case studies and practical applications, healthcare professionals will be better equipped to make informed decisions about nutrition therapy, improve the quality of nutritional care provided and achieve positive health outcomes for their patients.

17.1 Analysis of concrete cases of therapeutic menu planning

Let's take a look at two concrete cases of therapeutic menu planning:

Case 1: Management of type 2 diabetes in an adult :

Patient: Mr. Smith, 55 years old, newly diagnosed with type diabetes 2

.

Initial assessment: Mr. Smith has a high BMI and a sedentary lifestyle. His medical history reveals hypertension. He regularly consumes meals rich in carbohydrates and saturated fats.

Nutritional targets :

1. Control blood sugar levels by regulating carbohydrate intake.
2. Encourage moderate weight loss to reduce insulin resistance.
3. Reduce sodium intake to manage hypertension.

Therapeutic menu plan :

- Breakfast: Vegetable omelette with sliced avocado.
- Lunch: Grilled chicken salad with olive oil vinaigrette, steamed green vegetables.
- Afternoon snack: Plain Greek yogurt with berries.
- Dinner: Baked fish with quinoa and roasted vegetables.
- Evening snack: Handful of unsalted nuts.

Justification:

- Meals are rich in protein and fiber, which helps control blood sugar levels and promote satiety.
- The healthy fats found in avocado and olive oil help regulate blood

sugar and reduce inflammation.

- Controlling portion sizes and limiting simple carbohydrates helps prevent blood sugar spikes.
- Reducing sodium intake helps manage high blood pressure.

Case 2: Management of hypertension in adults :

Patient: Mrs Johnson, 65, with uncontrolled hypertension.

Initial assessment: Mrs. Johnson has a normal BMI but has a high sodium intake and a low potassium intake. She regularly consumes processed foods and fast foods.

Nutritional targets :

1. Reduce sodium intake to control blood pressure.
2. Increase potassium intake to promote cardiovascular health.
3. Encourage a balanced diet low in saturated fats.

Therapeutic menu plan :

- Breakfast: Oat flakes cooked in almond milk, topped with sliced bananas and walnuts.
- Lunch: Grilled chicken sandwich on whole-wheat bread with spinach and tomato salad.
- Afternoon snack: Fresh vegetables with hummus.
- Dinner: Steamed fish with brown rice and steamed vegetables.
- Evening snack: Plain Greek yogurt with kiwi slices.

Justification:

- Foods rich in potassium, such as bananas, vegetables and low-fat dairy products, help lower blood pressure.

- Limiting sodium-rich foods such as processed foods and ready-made meals helps reduce blood pressure.
- The healthy fats in nuts and avocado contribute to cardiovascular health.

In both cases, menu planning is tailored to patients' specific needs to help manage their underlying medical conditions while promoting a balanced, nutritious diet.

17.2 Development of therapeutic menus for different populations and medical conditions

Developing therapeutic menus tailored to different populations and medical conditions requires a personalized approach based on specific nutritional needs and treatment goals. Here are details and examples for several common populations and medical conditions:

1. Type 2 diabetes in adults:

- Nutritional targets :

Control blood sugar levels, promote weight loss, reduce the risk of cardiovascular complications.

- Sample menu: Breakfast: Vegetable omelette. Lunch: Quinoa salad with black beans. Dinner: Grilled salmon with broccoli and sweet potatoes.

2. Hypertension in the elderly:

- Nutritional targets :

Reduce sodium intake, increase potassium intake, promote

cardiovascular health.

- Sample menu: Breakfast: Oatmeal with berries and almonds. Lunch: Turkey sandwich on wholemeal bread with cucumber and tomato salad. Dinner: Roast chicken with sweet potatoes and green beans.

3. Chronic kidney disease :

- Nutritional targets :

Limit protein, phosphorus and potassium intake, control blood pressure.

- Sample menu: Breakfast: Fruit smoothie with almond milk. Lunch: Grilled chicken salad with avocado and green vegetables. Dinner: Poached white fish with white rice and asparagus.

4. Weight management for adolescents:

- Nutritional objectives: Encourage a balanced diet, promote physical activity, avoid restrictive diets.
- Sample menu: Breakfast: Greek yoghurt with granola and fresh fruit. Lunch: Grilled chicken and vegetable wrap with crudité and hummus. Dinner: Zucchini spaghetti with homemade tomato sauce and lean meatballs.

5. Celiac disease in children:

- Nutritional targets :

Eliminate gluten, ensure adequate nutrient intake, avoid cross-contamination. - Sample menu: Breakfast: Millet flakes cooked in almond milk with fruit. Lunch: Gluten-free ham and lettuce sandwich on corn bread. Dinner: Grilled chicken with quinoa and sautéed vegetables.

6. Cancer under treatment :

- Nutritional objectives: Maintain a stable body weight, prevent malnutrition, support the immune system.
- Sample menu: Breakfast: Protein smoothie with spinach and berries. Lunch: Chicken salad with avocado and sunflower seeds. Dinner: Baked fish with sweet potatoes and broccoli.

By developing therapeutic menus specific to each population and medical condition, it is possible to meet the unique nutritional needs of individuals while promoting their overall health and well-being.

17.3 Presentations of practical experience in preparing and implementing therapeutic menus

Presenting practical experiences in the preparation and implementation of therapeutic menus offers valuable insight into the challenges encountered and the best practices developed to overcome these challenges. Here are some details and examples based on real-life experiences:

1. Therapeutic nutrition management in a long-term care facility :

- Experience: At a long-term care center, a multidisciplinary team including dieticians, nurses and chefs collaborated to develop menus adapted to the needs of residents, many of whom suffered from medical conditions such as diabetes, hypertension and dysphagia.
- Details: Menus have been designed to offer balanced meals, adapted to the individual dietary restrictions and specific medical needs of each resident. Strategies have been put in place to accommodate dietary preferences and ensure residents' food safety, taking into

account appropriate textures for those with swallowing difficulties.

- Example: The menu included low-sodium options, sugar-free alternatives for desserts, as well as blended or chopped meals for residents with swallowing problems.

2. Therapeutic nutrition program in a dietetic consulting room:

- Experience: A dietary consulting practice has set up a therapeutic nutrition program for patients with metabolic diseases such as diabetes and hypercholesterolemia.
- Details: Dieticians developed personalized menus for each patient, taking into account their specific nutritional needs, food preferences and lifestyle. Individual counseling sessions were organized to educate patients on managing their diets, including reading nutrition labels, meal planning and managing social situations.
- Example: A diabetic patient benefited from a therapeutic nutrition program involving a reduction in simple carbohydrate intake, an increase in dietary fiber and a balanced distribution of meals throughout the day. The patient was encouraged to include a variety of low-glycemic index foods in his daily diet, and to monitor his blood glucose regularly to assess progress.

3. Therapeutic nutrition initiative in a community health clinic :

- Experience: A community health clinic launched a therapeutic nutrition initiative for community members at risk of cardiovascular disease.
- Details: Educational workshops were organized to teach participants the principles of healthy, balanced eating, as well as

practical strategies for implementing these changes in their daily lives. Cooking demonstration sessions were offered to show participants how to prepare healthy and tasty meals at home, using affordable and readily available ingredients.

- Example: A participant in the initiative learned how to prepare meals based on whole grains, lean proteins and colorful vegetables. By following the nutritional advice provided at the workshops, the participant was able to reduce his weight, improve his lipid profile and lower his blood pressure.

By sharing these practical experiences, healthcare professionals can benefit from the lessons learned and effective strategies developed to deliver quality therapeutic nutrition to individuals in a variety of healthcare settings.

CONCLUSION

In conclusion, the "Guide Pratique de la Nutrition en Milieu de Soins en République Démocratique du Congo : Préparation des Menus et Aliments Thérapeutiques" is an indispensable resource for all those striving to ensure adequate, therapeutic nutrition for patients in Congolese healthcare establishments. Its information-rich content and practical advice make it an invaluable tool for promoting the health and well-being of populations in the specific context of the DRC.

APPENDIX: PROSPECTS FOR THE FUTURE OF HEALTHCARE NUTRITION IN THE DEMOCRATIC REPUBLIC OF CONGO

The outlook for the future of healthcare nutrition in the Democratic Republic of Congo is promising, but requires continued attention and concerted efforts. Here are some key prospects for improving nutrition in care facilities in the DRC:

1. **Strengthening infrastructure and human resources:** investing in the improvement of infrastructure and human resources in healthcare facilities is essential to guarantee quality nutritional services. This includes training and upskilling healthcare staff, as well as improving equipment and kitchen facilities.
2. **Integrating nutrition into public health policies:** integrating nutrition into public health policies is necessary to ensure that nutrition is a priority in national health programs. This involves developing and implementing policies to promote healthy eating, prevent malnutrition and improve the quality of nutritional care.
3. **Promotion of breastfeeding and infant nutrition:** the promotion of exclusive breastfeeding and appropriate infant nutrition is crucial to preventing malnutrition in infants and young children. Awareness-raising and support initiatives need to be developed to encourage optimal breastfeeding and dietary diversification practices.
4. **Intersectoral collaboration:** nutrition is an area that requires an intersectoral approach, involving collaboration between the health sector, agriculture, education and other relevant sectors. By fostering

collaboration and coordination between these different players, it is possible to develop holistic solutions to improve nutrition in the country.

5. **Research and innovation:** research and innovation are essential for advancing understanding of the DRC's nutritional challenges and developing effective interventions to address them. There is a need to invest in nutrition research, including operational research and the implementation of pilot studies to assess the effectiveness of interventions.

By implementing these perspectives for the future, the Democratic Republic of Congo can move towards more nutritious and holistic healthcare, improving the health and well-being of its population.

BIBLIOGRAPHICAL REFERENCES

- **American Diabetes Association. (2019).** American Diabetes Association Diabetes Cookbook (2nd ed.). Alexandria, VA: American Diabetes Association.
- **American Heart Association. (2017**). American Heart Association Healthy Fats, LowCholesterol Cookbook: Delicious Recipes to Help Reduce Bad Fats and Lower Your Cholesterol. New York, NY: Harmony.
- **Elsevier.Thomas, B., Bishop, J., & Beller, E. M. (2013).** Texture-Modified Food for Improving the Oral Intake of Older Adults in Long-Term Care Facilities: A Systematic Review. Journal of the American Medical Directors Association, 14(2), 119-130. https: //doi.org/ 10.1016/j.jamda.2012.08.006
- **Escott-Stump, S. (2012).** Nutrition and Diagnosis-Related Care (7th ed.). Philadelphia, PA: Lippincott Williams & Wilkins.
- **Heller, M. (2012).** The DASH Diet Action Plan: Proven to Lower Blood Pressure and Cholesterol without Medication. New York, NY: Grand Central Life & Style.
- **Katz, D. L., & Meller, S. (2014).** Can We Say What Diet Is Best for Health? Annual Review of Public Health, 35(1), 83-103. https://doi.org/10.1146/annurev-publhealth-032013-182351 **Kopple, J. D., & National Kidney Foundation. (2013**). National Kidney Foundation Primer on Kidney Diseases (6th ed.). Philadelphia, PA: Elsevier/Saunders.
- **Krause, M. V., Mahan, L. K., & Escott-Stump, S. (2017).** Food, Nutrition, & Diet Therapy (14th ed.). St. Louis, MO: Elsevier.

- **Lee, R. D., & Nieman, D. C. (2018).** Nutritional Assessment (7th ed.). New York: McGrawHill Education.
- **Mahan, L. K., & Raymond, J. L. (2016**). Krause's Food & the Nutrition Care Process (14th ed.). St. Louis, MO: Elsevier.
- Satia, J. A. (2010). Dietary Acculturation and the Nutrition Transition: An Overview. Applied Physiology, Nutrition, and Metabolism, 35(2), 219-223. https://doi.org/10.1139/H10-007
- Sobal, J. (2001). Food System Globalization, Eating Transformations, and Nutrition Transitions. In M. Douglas & S. L. Mical (Eds.), Food Matters: Perspectives on an Emerging Field (pp. 99-114). Ithaca, NY: Cornell University Press.
- **Sullivan, S. (2016).** Kidney Health Gourmet Diet Guide & Cookbook. CreateSpace Independent Publishing Platform.
- **Williams, L. (2019**). Essentials of Nutrition and Diet Therapy (12th ed.). St. Louis, MO:
- Elsevier.
- **Whitney, E., Rolfes, S. R., Crowe, T., & Cameron-Smith, D. (2016).** Understanding
- Nutrition: Australian and New Zealand Edition (2nd ed.). South Melbourne, VIC: Cengage Learning Australia.

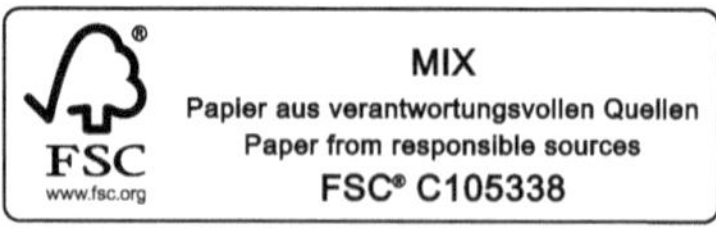

Printed by Books on Demand GmbH, Norderstedt / Germany